Brain Death & Disorders of Consciousness

Contents

1 Introduction to Brain Death & Disorders of Consciousness   **1**

   1.1   Brain death 1

       1.1.1   Legal history 1

       1.1.2   Medical criteria 2

       1.1.3   Organ donation 2

       1.1.4   See also 3

       1.1.5   References 3

   1.2   Disorders of consciousness 4

       1.2.1   Classification 4

       1.2.2   See also 5

       1.2.3   References 5

2 Brain Death & Disorders of Consciousness Articles   **6**

   2.1   Brain stem death 6

       2.1.1   Evolution of diagnostic criteria 6

       2.1.2   Diagnosis 7

       2.1.3   Prognosis and management 7

       2.1.4   Criticism 7

       2.1.5   References 8

       2.1.6   External links 9

   2.2   Caloric reflex test 9

       2.2.1   Utility 9

       2.2.2   Technique and results 9

       2.2.3   Mnemonic 10

       2.2.4   See also 10

       2.2.5   References 10

   2.3   Clinical death 10

       2.3.1   Limits of reversal 11

       2.3.2   Hypothermia during clinical death 11

       2.3.3   Life support during clinical death 11

2.3.4   Controlled clinical death   12

2.3.5   Clinical death and the determination of death   12

2.3.6   See also   12

2.3.7   References   12

2.4   Coma   14

2.4.1   Signs and symptoms   14

2.4.2   Diagnosis   15

2.4.3   Treatment   17

2.4.4   Prognosis   18

2.4.5   Society and culture   18

2.4.6   See also   18

2.4.7   References   19

2.5   Corneal reflex   19

2.5.1   Rates   20

2.5.2   See also   20

2.5.3   References   20

2.5.4   External links   20

2.6   Do not resuscitate   20

2.6.1   Alternative terms   21

2.6.2   Usage by country   21

2.6.3   See also   22

2.6.4   References   22

2.6.5   External links   23

2.7   Electroencephalography   23

2.7.1   Medical use   23

2.7.2   Research use   25

2.7.3   Mechanisms   26

2.7.4   Method   27

2.7.5   Normal activity   29

2.7.6   Artifacts   31

2.7.7   Abnormal activity   32

2.7.8   Economics   33

2.7.9   History   34

2.7.10   Future research   34

2.7.11   See also   35

2.7.12   References   35

2.7.13   Further reading   39

2.7.14   External links   39

2.8   Information-theoretic death 39

    2.8.1   References 40

    2.8.2   External links 40

2.9   Lazarus sign 40

    2.9.1   How it happens 40

    2.9.2   Occurrences 41

    2.9.3   See also 41

    2.9.4   References 41

2.10   Legal death 41

    2.10.1   Medical declaration 41

    2.10.2   Presumption of death 41

    2.10.3   Fraudulent death 41

    2.10.4   Investigation 41

    2.10.5   Estate 42

    2.10.6   Reversal 42

    2.10.7   References 42

2.11   Life support 42

    2.11.1   Bioethics 42

    2.11.2   Techniques 43

    2.11.3   Gallery 43

    2.11.4   References 43

2.12   Locked-in syndrome 43

    2.12.1   Presentation 43

    2.12.2   Causes 44

    2.12.3   Diagnosis 44

    2.12.4   Treatment 44

    2.12.5   Prognosis 44

    2.12.6   Research 44

    2.12.7   See also 44

    2.12.8   References 45

    2.12.9   Further reading 45

    2.12.10 External links 45

2.13   Mechanical ventilation 45

    2.13.1   Medical uses 46

    2.13.2   Associated risk 46

    2.13.3   Application and duration 47

    2.13.4   Types of ventilators 48

    2.13.5   Breath delivery 49

2.13.6   Breath exhalation   49

2.13.7   Dead space   49

2.13.8   Modes of ventilation   49

2.13.9   Modification of settings   49

2.13.10 Respiratory monitoring   50

2.13.11 Artificial airways as a connection to the ventilator   50

2.13.12 Ventilation formulas   51

2.13.13 History   51

2.13.14 References   51

2.13.15 External links   52

2.14   Minimally conscious state   52

2.14.1   History   52

2.14.2   Definition and diagnostic criteria   52

2.14.3   Prognosis   53

2.14.4   Pathophysiology   53

2.14.5   Treatment   55

2.14.6   Ethical issues   55

2.14.7   Notable patients   56

2.14.8   References   56

2.15   Organ donation   57

2.15.1   Legislation and global perspectives   57

2.15.2   Iran   61

2.15.3   Bioethical issues   61

2.15.4   Political issues   63

2.15.5   Religious viewpoints   64

2.15.6   Organ shortfall   65

2.15.7   Distribution   66

2.15.8   Suicide   66

2.15.9   Controversies   66

2.15.10 Social media   67

2.15.11 Becoming a donor   67

2.15.12 Public service announcements   67

2.15.13 See also   68

2.15.14 References   68

2.15.15 External links   72

2.16   Persistent vegetative state   72

2.16.1   Definition   72

2.16.2   Signs and symptoms   73

2.16.3 Causes 74

2.16.4 Diagnosis 74

2.16.5 Treatment 76

2.16.6 Epidemiology 76

2.16.7 History 76

2.16.8 Society and culture 76

2.16.9 See also 77

2.16.10 Notes 77

2.16.11 References 78

2.16.12 Further reading 79

2.17 Pupillary reflex 79

2.17.1 References 79

2.18 Unconsciousness 79

2.18.1 Law and medicine 80

2.18.2 See also 80

2.18.3 References 80

2.19 Uniform Determination of Death Act 80

2.19.1 Section 1 80

2.19.2 Section 2 81

2.19.3 See also 81

2.19.4 External links 81

2.20 Vegetative symptoms 81

2.20.1 Reversed vegetative symptoms 81

2.20.2 See also 81

2.20.3 References 81

2.21 Vestibulo–ocular reflex 81

2.21.1 Circuit 82

2.21.2 Speed 83

2.21.3 Gain 83

2.21.4 Testing 83

2.21.5 Role of cerebellum 83

2.21.6 See also 84

2.21.7 References 84

2.21.8 External links 84

3 Text and image sources, contributors, and licenses   85

3.1 Text 85

3.2 Images 90

3.3 Content license 92

Chapter 1

Introduction to Brain Death & Disorders of Consciousness

1.1 Brain death

For the EP by Nuclear Assault, see Brain Death (EP). "Brain-dead" redirects here. For other uses, see Brain Dead.

Brain death is the complete and irreversible loss of brain function (including involuntary activity necessary to sustain life).[1][2][3][4] Brain death is one of the two ways of determination of death, according to the Uniform Determination of Death Act of the United States (the other way of determining death being "irreversible cessation of circulatory and respiratory functions").[5] It is not the same as persistent vegetative state, in which the person is "alive".

Brain death is used as an indicator of legal death in many jurisdictions, but it is defined inconsistently. Various parts of the brain may keep living when others die, and the term "brain death" has been used to refer to various combinations. For example, although a major medical dictionary[6] says that "brain death" is synonymous with "cerebral death" (death of the cerebrum), the US National Library of Medicine Medical Subject Headings (MeSH) system defines brain death as including the brainstem. The distinctions can be important because, for example, in someone with a dead cerebrum but a living brainstem, the heartbeat and ventilation can continue unaided, whereas in whole-brain death (which includes brain stem death), only life support equipment would keep those functions going. Patients classified as brain-dead can have their organs surgically removed for organ donation; though not everyone agrees with this practice, preferring to limit organ donation to those individuals who have suffered the death of all of their brain and the death of their cardiac and respiratory systems (biological, or full, death). However, if one limits the criteria to those individuals, procuring viable organs can become much more difficult.

1.1.1 Legal history

Traditionally, both the legal and medical communities determined death through the permanent end of certain bodily functions in clinical death, especially respiration and heartbeat. With the increasing ability of the medical community to resuscitate people with no respiration, heartbeat, or other external signs of life, the need for another definition of death occurred, raising questions of legal death. This gained greater urgency with the widespread use of life support equipment, as well as rising capabilities and demand for organ transplantation.

Since the 1960s, laws on determining death have, therefore, been implemented in all countries with active organ transplantation programs. The first European country to adopt brain death as a legal definition (or indicator) of death was Finland, in 1971. In the United States, Kansas had enacted a similar law earlier.[7] In the 1970s, the Supreme Court of the state of New Jersey ruled that patients and their families have the right to decide when and whether to remove life support.[8]

An *ad hoc* committee at Harvard Medical School published a pivotal 1968 report to define irreversible coma.[9][10] The Harvard criteria gradually gained consensus toward what is now known as brain death. In the wake of the 1976 Karen Ann Quinlan controversy, state legislatures in the United States moved to accept brain death as an acceptable indication of death. In 1981 a Presidential commission issued a landmark report – *Defining Death: Medical, Legal, and Ethical Issues in the Determination of Death* [11] – that rejected the "higher brain" approach to death in favor of a "whole brain" definition. This report was the basis for the Uniform Determination of Death Act, which has been enacted in 39 states of the United States[12] the Uniform Determination of Death Act in the United States attempts to standardize criteria. Today, both the legal and medical communities in the US use "brain death" as a legal definition of death, allowing a person to be declared legally dead even if life support equipment keeps the body's metabolic processes working.

In the UK, the Royal College of Physicians reported in 1995, abandoning the 1979 claim that the tests published in 1976 sufficed for the diagnosis of brain death and suggesting a new definition of death based on the irreversible loss of brain stem function alone.[13] This new definition, the irreversible loss of the capacity for consciousness and for spontaneous breathing, and the essentially unchanged 1976 tests held to establish that state, have been adopted as a basis of death certification for organ transplant purposes in subsequent Codes of Practice.[14][15]

1.1.2 Medical criteria

It is very important for family members and health care professionals to be aware of natural movements also known as Lazarus sign or Lazarus reflex, that can occur on a brain-dead person whose organs have been kept functioning by life support. The living cells that can cause these movements, are not living cells from the brain, or brain stem these cells come from the spinal cord. Sometimes these body movements can cause false hope for the family members.

A brain-dead individual has no clinical evidence of brain function upon physical examination. This includes no response to pain and no cranial nerve reflexes. Reflexes include pupillary response (fixed pupils), oculocephalic reflex, corneal reflex, no response to the caloric reflex test, and no spontaneous respirations.

It is important to distinguish between brain death and states that may be difficult to differentiate from brain death (such as barbiturate overdose, alcohol intoxication, sedative overdose, hypothermia, hypoglycemia, coma, and chronic vegetative states). Some comatose patients can recover to pre-coma or near pre-coma level of functioning, and some patients with severe irreversible neurological dysfunction will nonetheless retain some lower brain functions such as spontaneous respiration, despite the losses of both cortex and brain stem functionality; such is the case with anencephaly.

Note that brain electrical activity can stop completely, or drop to such a low level as to be undetectable with most equipment. An EEG will therefore be flat, though this is sometimes also observed during deep anesthesia or cardiac arrest.[16] Although in the United States a flat EEG test is not required to certify death, it is considered to have confirmatory value. In the UK it is not considered to be of value because any continuing activity it might reveal in parts of the brain above the brain stem is held to be irrelevant to the diagnosis of death on the Code of Practice criteria.[17]

The diagnosis of brain death needs to be rigorous, in order

to be certain that the condition is irreversible. Legal criteria vary, but in general they require neurological examinations by two independent physicians. The exams must show complete and irreversible absence of brain function (brain stem function in UK),[18] and may include two isoelectric (flatline) EEGs 24 hours apart (less in other countries where it is accepted that if the cause of the dysfunction is a clear physical trauma there is no need to wait that long to establish irreversibility). The patient should have a normal temperature and be free of drugs that can suppress brain activity if the diagnosis is to be made on EEG criteria.

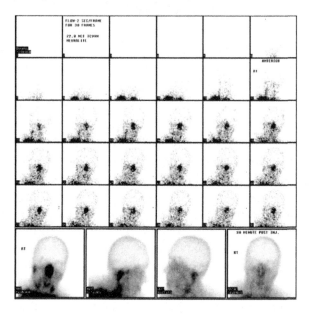

Radionuclide scan: No intracranial blood flow and "hot-nose" sign.

Also, a radionuclide cerebral blood flow scan that shows complete absence of intracranial blood flow must be considered with other exams – temporary swelling of the brain, particularly within the first 72 hours, can lead to a false positive test on a patient that may recover with more time.[19] Zack Dunlap in 2008 had a false positive of this type, likely due to temporary cerebral edema.

CT angiography is neither required nor sufficient test to make the diagnosis.[20]

1.1.3 Organ donation

Main article: Organ donation

While the diagnosis of brain death has become accepted as a basis for the certification of death for legal purposes, it should be clearly understood that it is a very different state from biological death - the state universally recognized and understood as death.[21] The continuing function of vital organs in the bodies of those diagnosed brain dead, if mechanical ventilation and other life-support measures are continued, provides optimal opportunities for their transplantation.

When mechanical ventilation is used to support the body of a brain dead organ donor pending a transplant into an organ recipient, the donor's date of death is listed as the date that brain death was diagnosed.[22]

In some countries (for instance, Spain,[23] Poland, Wales, Portugal, and France), everyone is automatically an organ donor after diagnosis of death on legally accepted criteria, although some jurisdictions (such as Singapore, Spain, Wales, France, Czech Republic and Portugal) allow opting out of the system. Elsewhere, consent from family members or next-of-kin may be required for organ donation. In New Zealand, Australia, United Kingdom (excluding Wales) and most states in the United States, drivers are asked upon application if they wish to be registered as an organ donor.[24]

In the United States, if the patient is at or near death, the hospital must notify a transplant organization of the person's details and maintain the patient while the patient is being evaluated for suitability as a donor.[25] The patient is kept on ventilator support until the organs have been surgically removed. If the patient has indicated in an advance health care directive that they do not wish to receive mechanical ventilation or has specified a do not resuscitate order and the patient has also indicated that they wish to donate their organs, some vital organs such as the heart and lungs may not be able to be recovered.[26]

1.1.4 See also

- Brainstem death
- Clinical death
- Death
- Persistent vegetative state
- Information-theoretic death
- Consciousness after death

1.1.5 References

[1] "Brain death". *Encyclopedia of Death and Dying*. Retrieved 25 March 2014.

[2] Young, G Bryan. "Diagnosis of brain death". *UpToDate*. Retrieved 25 March 2014.

[3] Goila, A.; Pawar, M. (2009). "The diagnosis of brain death". *Indian Journal of Critical Care Medicine* **13** (1): 7–11. doi:10.4103/0972-5229.53108. PMC 2772257. PMID 19881172.

[4] Machado, C. (2010). "Diagnosis of brain death". *Neurology International* **2**. doi:10.4081/ni.2010.e2.

[5] "Uniform Determination of Death Act" (PDF). National Conference of Commissioners on Uniform State Laws. Retrieved 26 March 2014.

[6] Elsevier, *Dorland's Illustrated Medical Dictionary*, Elsevier.

[7] (Randell T. (2004). "Medical and legal considerations of brain death". *Acta Anaesthesiologica Scandinavica* **48** (2): 139–144. doi:10.1111/j.0001-5172.2004.00304.x. PMID 14995934.

[8] Epstein, Sue (April 28, 2010). "N.J. court to rule whether hospitals may refuse life support despite wishes of families, patients". NJ.com. Retrieved March 5, 2014.

[9] "A definition of irreversible coma: report of the Ad Hoc Committee of the Harvard Medical School to Examine the Definition of Brain Death". *JAMA* **205**: 337–40. 1968. doi:10.1001/jama.1968.03140320031009.

[10] Life-sustaining Technologies and the Elderly

[11] "Defining death: a report on the medical, legal and ethical issues in the determination of death".

[12] "Legislative Fact Sheet – Determination of Death Act". Uniform Law Commission. Retrieved 8 May 2012.

[13] Criteria for the diagnosis of brain stem death. J Roy Coll Physns of London 1995;29:381-2

[14] A Code of Practice for the Diagnosis and Confirmation of Death. Academy of Medical Royal Colleges. 70 Wimpole Street, London, 2008

[15] American Academy of Neurology. (2000, January 13).Spontaneous Movements Often Occur After Brain Death.Science Daily.

[16] Karasawa, H; et al. (Jan 2001). "Intracranial electroencephalographic changes in deep anesthesia". *Clin Neurophysiol* **112** (1): 25–30. doi:10.1016/s1388-2457(00)00510-1. PMID 11137657.

[17] A Code of Practice for the Diagnosis of Death. Academy of Medical Royal Colleges, 70 Wimpole Street, London, 2008

[18] Waters, C. E.; French, G.; Burt, M. "Difficulty in brainstem death testing in the presence of high spinal cord injury". *British Journal of Anaesthesia* **92** (5): 762. doi:10.1093/bja/aeh117.

[19] http://theness.com/neurologicablog/index.php/brain-dead/

[20] Taylor, T; Dineen, RA; Gardiner, DC; Buss, CH; Howatson, A; Pace, NL (Mar 31, 2014). "Computed tomography (CT) angiography for confirmation of the clinical diagnosis of brain death.". *The Cochrane database of systematic reviews* **3**: CD009694. doi:10.1002/14651858.CD009694.pub2. PMID 24683063.

[21] Truog RD, Miller FG. The meaning of brain death. JAMA Internal Medicine 2014, Publ online June 9, 2014 : http://archinte.jamanetwork.com

[22] "Understanding Brain Death". What is the legal time of death for a brain dead patient? The legal time of death is the date and time that doctors determine that all brain activity has ceased. This is the time that is noted on the patient's death certificate.

[23] Organización Nacional de Transplantes – Consentimiento familiar y donación

[24] "National Donate Life America Donor Designation State Report Card 2013" (PDF). pp. 6 & 7. 2012 State Comparisons

[25] "State and Federal Law on Organ Procurement". Unless the individual expressed contrary intent, a hospital must take measures to ensure the medical suitability of an individual at or near death while a procurement organization examines the patient for suitability as a donor.

[26] "Frequently Asked Questions About Donation". DNR will be honored. You can still be a tissue donor.

1.2   Disorders of consciousness

Disorders of consciousness are medical conditions that inhibit consciousness.[1] Some define disorders of consciousness as any change from complete self-awareness to inhibited or absent self-awareness. This category generally includes minimally conscious state and persistent vegetative state, but sometimes also includes the less severe locked-in syndrome and more severe chronic coma.[1][2] Differential diagnosis of these disorders is an active area of biomedical research.[3][4][5] Finally, brain death results in an irreversible disruption of consciousness.[1] While other conditions may cause a moderate deterioration (e.g., dementia and delirium) or transient interruption (e.g., grand mal and petit mal seizures) of consciousness, they are not included in this category.

1.2.1   Classification

Locked-in syndrome

Main article: Locked-in syndrome

In locked-in syndrome the patient has awareness, sleep-wake cycles, and meaningful behavior (viz., eye-movement), but is isolated due to quadriplegia and pseudobulbar palsy. Locked-in syndrome is a condition in which a patient is aware and awake but cannot move or communicate verbally due to complete paralysis of nearly all voluntary muscles in the body except for the eyes. Total locked-in syndrome is a version of locked-in syndrome where the eyes are paralyzed as well.[6]

Minimally conscious state

Main article: Minimally conscious state

In a minimally conscious state, the patient has intermittent periods of awareness and wakefulness and displays some meaningful behavior.

Persistent vegetative state

Main article: Persistent vegetative state

In a persistent vegetative state, the patient has sleep-wake cycles, but lacks awareness and only displays reflexive and non-purposeful behavior. It is a diagnosis of some uncertainty in that it deals with a syndrome. After four weeks in a vegetative state (VS), the patient is classified as in a persistent vegetative state. This diagnosis is classified as a permanent vegetative state (PVS) after approximately 1 year of being in a vegetative state.

Chronic coma

Main article: Chronic coma

In chronic coma the patient lacks awareness and sleep-wake cycles and only displays reflexive behavior. In medicine, a coma (from the Greek κῶμα koma, meaning deep sleep) is a state of unconsciousness, lasting more than six hours in which a person cannot be awakened, fails to respond normally to painful stimuli, light, sound, lacks a normal sleep-wake cycle and does not initiate voluntary actions. A person in a state of coma is described as comatose. Although, according to the Glasgow Coma Scale, a person with confusion is considered to be in the mildest coma.

Although a coma patient may appear to be awake, they are unable to consciously feel, speak, hear, or move. For a patient to maintain consciousness, two important neurological components must function impeccably. The first is the cerebral cortex which is the gray matter covering the outer layer of the brain. The other is a structure located in the brainstem, called reticular activating system (RAS or ARAS). Injury to either or both of these components is sufficient to cause a patient to experience a coma.

Brain death

Main article: Brain death

Brain death is the irreversible end of all brain activity, and function (including involuntary activity necessary to sustain life). The main cause is total necrosis of the cerebral neurons following loss of brain oxygenation. After brain death the patient lacks any sense of awareness; sleep-wake cycles or behavior, and typically look as if they are dead or are in a deep sleep-state or coma. Although visually similar to a comatose state such as persistent vegetative state, the two should not be confused. Patients classified as brain dead are legally dead and can qualify as organ donors, in which their organs are surgically removed and prepared for a particular recipient.

Brain death is one of the deciding factors when pronouncing a trauma patient as dead. Determining function and presence of necrosis after trauma to the whole brain or brainstem may be used to determine brain death, and is used in many states in the US.

1.2.2 See also

- Neuropsychology

- Neuropsychological assessment

1.2.3 References

[1] Bernat JL (8 Apr 2006). "Chronic disorders of consciousness". *Lancet* **367** (9517): 1181–1192. doi:10.1016/S0140-6736(06)68508-5. PMID 16616561.

[2] Bernat JL (20 Jul 2010). "The natural history of chronic disorders of consciousness". *Neurol* **75** (3): 206–207. doi:10.1212/WNL.0b013e3181e8e960. PMID 20554939.

[3] Coleman MR, Davis MH, Rodd JM, Robson T, Ali A, Owen AM, Pickard JD (Sep 2009). "Towards the routine use of brain imaging to aid the clinical diagnosis of disorders of consciousness". *Brain* **132** (9): 2541–2552. doi:10.1093/brain/awp183. PMID 19710182.

[4] Monti MM, Vanhaudenhuyse A, Coleman MR, Boly M, Pickard JD, Tshibanda L, Owen AM, Laureys S (18 Feb 2010). "Willful modulation of brain activity in disorders of consciousness". *N Engl J Med* **362** (7): 579–589. doi:10.1056/NEJMoa0905370. PMID 20130250.

[5] Seel RT, Sherer M, Whyte J, Katz DI, Giacino JT, Rosenbaum AM, Hammond FM, Kalmar K, Pape TL et al. (Dec 2010). "Assessment scales for disorders of consciousness: evidence-based recommendations for clinical practice and research". *Arch Phys Med Rehabil* **91** (12): 1795–1813. doi:10.1016/j.apmr.2011.01.002. PMID 21112421.

[6] Bauer, G. and Gerstenbrand, F. and Rumpl, E. (1979). "Varieties of the locked-in syndrome". *Journal of Neurology* **221** (2): 77–91. doi:10.1007/BF00313105. PMID 92545.

Chapter 2

Brain Death & Disorders of Consciousness Articles

2.1 Brain stem death

Brain stem death is a clinical syndrome defined by the absence of reflexes with pathways through the brain stem - the "stalk" of the brain, which connects the spinal cord to the mid-brain, cerebellum and cerebral hemispheres - in a deeply comatose, ventilator-dependent patient. Identification of this state carries a very grave prognosis for survival; cessation of heartbeat often occurs within a few days although it may continue for weeks or even months if intensive support is maintained.[1]

In the United Kingdom, the formal diagnosis of brain stem death by the procedure laid down in the official Code of Practice[1] permits the diagnosis and certification of death on the premise that a person is dead when consciousness and the ability to breathe are permanently lost, regardless of continuing life in the body and parts of the brain, and that death of the brain stem alone is sufficient to produce this state.[2]

This concept of brain stem death is also accepted as grounds for pronoucing death for legal purposes in India[3] and Trinidad & Tobago.[4] Elsewhere in the world the concept upon which the certification of death on neurological grounds is based is that of permanent cessation of all function in all parts of the brain - whole brain death - with which the reductionist United Kingdom concept should not be confused. The United States' President's Council on Bioethics made it clear, in its White Paper of December 2008, that the United Kingdom concept and clinical criteria are not considered sufficient for the diagnosis of death in the United States of America.[5]

2.1.1 Evolution of diagnostic criteria

The United Kingdom (UK) criteria were first published by the Conference of Medical Royal Colleges (with advice from the Transplant Advisory Panel) in 1976, as prognostic guidelines.[6] They were drafted in response to a perceived need for guidance in the management of deeply comatose patients with severe brain damage who were being kept alive by mechanical ventilators but showing no signs of recovery. The Conference sought "to establish diagnostic criteria of such rigour that on their fulfilment the mechanical ventilator can be switched off, in the secure knowledge that there is no possible chance of recovery". The published criteria – negative responses to bedside tests of some reflexes with pathways through the brain stem and a specified challenge to the brain stem respiratory centre, with caveats about exclusion of endocrine influences, metabolic factors and drug effects – were held to be "sufficient to distinguish between those patients who retain the functional capacity to have a chance of even partial recovery and those where no such possibility exists". Recognition of that state required the withdrawal of fruitless further artificial support so that death might be allowed to occur, thus "sparing relatives from the further emotional trauma of sterile hope".[6]

In 1979, the Conference of Medical Royal Colleges promulgated its conclusion that identification of the state defined by those same criteria – then thought sufficient for a diagnosis of brain death – "means that the patient is dead" [7] Death certification on those criteria has continued in the United Kingdom (where there is no statutory legal definition of death) since that time, particularly for organ transplantation purposes, although the conceptual basis for that use has changed.

In 1995, after a review by a Working Group of the Royal College of Physicians of London, the Conference of Medical Royal Colleges [2] formally adopted the "more correct" term for the syndrome, "brain stem death" - championed by Pallis in a set of 1982 articles in the British Medical Journal [8] – and advanced a new definition of human death as the basis for equating this syndrome with the death of the person. The suggested new definition of death was the "irreversible loss of the capacity for consciousness, combined with irreversible loss of the capacity to breathe". It was stated that the irreversible cessation of brain stem function will produce this state and "therefore brain stem death is equivalent to the death of the individual".[2]

2.1.2 Diagnosis

In the UK, the formal rules for the diagnosis of brain stem death have undergone only minor modifications since they were first published [6] in 1976. The most recent revision of the UK's Department of Health Code of Practice governing use of that procedure for the diagnosis of death [1] reaffirms the preconditions for its consideration. These are:

1. There should be no doubt that the patient's condition – deeply comatose, unresponsive and requiring artificial ventilation – is due to irreversible brain damage of known aetiology.

2. There should be no evidence that this state is due to depressant drugs.

3. Primary hypothermia as the cause of unconsciousness must have been excluded, and

4. Potentially reversible circulatory, metabolic and endocrine disturbances likewise.

5. Potentially reversible causes of apnoea (dependence on the ventilator), such as muscle relaxants and cervical cord injury, must be excluded.

With these pre-conditions satisfied, the definitive criteria are:

1. Fixed pupils which do not respond to sharp changes in the intensity of incident light.

2. No corneal reflex.

3. Absent oculovestibular reflexes – no eye movements following the slow injection of at least 50ml of ice-cold water into each ear in turn (the caloric reflex test).

4. No response to supraorbital pressure.

5. No cough reflex to bronchial stimulation or gagging response to pharyngeal stimulation.

6. No observed respiratory effort in response to disconnection of the ventilator for long enough (typically 5 minutes) to ensure elevation of the arterial partial pressure of carbon dioxide to at least 6.0 kPa (6.5 kPa in patients with chronic carbon dioxide retention). Adequate oxygenation is ensured by pre-oxygenation and diffusion oxygenation during the disconnection (so the brain stem respiratory centre is not challenged

by the ultimate, anoxic, drive stimulus). This test - the apnoea test - is dangerous – and may prove lethal.[9][10][11][12]

Two doctors, of specified status and experience, are required to act together to diagnose death on these criteria and the tests must be repeated after "a short period of time ... to allow return of the patient's arterial blood gases and baseline parameters to the pre-test state". These criteria for the diagnosis of death are not applicable to infants below the age of two months

2.1.3 Prognosis and management

With due regard for the cause of the coma, and the rapidity of its onset, testing for the purpose of diagnosing death on brain stem death grounds may be delayed beyond the stage where brain stem reflexes may be absent only temporarily – because the cerebral blood flow is inadequate to support synaptic function although there is still sufficient blood flow to keep brain cells alive [9] and capable of recovery. There has recently been renewed interest in the possibility of neuronal protection during this phase by use of moderate hypothermia and by correction of the neuroendocrine abnormalities commonly seen in this early stage.[13]

Published studies of patients meeting the criteria for brain stem death or whole brain death – the American standard which includes brain stem death diagnosed by similar means – record that even if ventilation is continued after diagnosis, the heart stops beating within only a few hours or days.[14] However, there have been some very long-term survivals[15] and it is noteworthy that expert management can maintain the bodily functions of pregnant 'brain dead' women for long enough to bring them to term.[16]

The management of patients pronounced dead on meeting the brain stem death criteria depends upon the reason for diagnosing death on that basis. If the intent is to take organs from the body for transplantation, the ventilator is reconnected and life-support measures are continued, perhaps intensified, with the addition of procedures designed to protect the wanted organs until they can be removed. Otherwise, the ventilator is left disconnected on confirmation of the lack of respiratory centre response.

2.1.4 Criticism

The diagnostic criteria were originally published for the purpose of identifying a clinical state associated with a fatal prognosis (see above). The change of use, in the UK, to criteria for the diagnosis of death itself was protested from the first.[17][18] The initial basis for the change of use was the claim that satisfaction of the criteria sufficed for the diagnosis of the death of the brain as a whole, despite the persistence of demonstrable activity in parts of the brain.[19] In 1995, that claim was abandoned[7] and the diagnosis of death (acceptable for legal purposes in the UK in the context of organ procurement for transplantation) by the specified testing of brain stem functions was based on a new definition of death, viz. the permanent loss of the capacity for consciousness and spontaneous breathing. There are doubts that this concept is generally understood and accepted and that the specified testing is stringent enough to determine that state. It is, however, associated with substantial risk of exacerbating the brain damage and even causing the death of the apparently dying patient so tested (see "the apnoea test" above). This raises ethical problems which seem not to have been addressed.

It has been argued that sound scientific support is lacking for the claim that the specified purely bedside tests have the power to diagnose true and total death of the brain stem, the necessary condition for the assumption of permanent loss of the intrinsically untestable consciousness-arousal function of those elements of the reticular formation which lie within the brain stem (there are elements also within the higher brain).[19] Knowledge of this arousal system is based upon the findings from animal experiments[20][21][22] as illuminated by pathological studies in humans.[23] The current neurological consensus is that the arousal of consciousness depends upon reticular components which reside in the midbrain, diencephalon and pons.[24][25] It is said that the midbrain reticular formation may be viewed as a driving centre for the higher structures, loss of which produces a state in which the cortex appears, on the basis of electroencephalographic (EEG) studies, to be awaiting the command or ability to function. The role of diencephalic (higher brain) involvement is stated to be uncertain and we are reminded that the arousal system is best regarded as a physiological rather than a precise anatomical entity. There should, perhaps, also be a caveat about possible arousal mechanisms involving the first and second cranial nerves (serving sight and smell) which are not tested when diagnosing brain stem death but which were described in cats in 1935 and 1938.[20] In humans, light flashes have been observed to disturb the sleep-like EEG activity persisting after the loss of all brain stem reflexes and of spontaneous respiration.[26]

There is also concern about the permanence of consciousness loss, based on studies in cats, dogs and monkeys which recovered consciousness days or weeks after being rendered comatose by brain stem ablation and on human studies of brain stem stroke raising thoughts about the "plasticity" of the nervous system.[23] Other theories of consciousness place more stress on the thalamocortical system.[27] Perhaps the most objective statement to be made is that consciousness is not currently understood. That being so, proper caution must be exercised in accepting a diagnosis of its permanent loss before all cerebral blood flow has permanently ceased.

The ability to breathe spontaneously depends upon functioning elements in the medulla – the 'respiratory centre'. In the UK, establishing a neurological diagnosis of death involves challenging this centre with the strong stimulus offered by an unusually high concentration of carbon dioxide in the arterial blood, but it is not challenged by the more powerful drive stimulus provided by anoxia – although the effect of that ultimate stimulus is sometimes seen after final disconnection of the ventilator in the form of agonal gasps.

No testing of testable brain stem functions such as oesophageal and cardiovascular regulation is specified in the UK Code of Practice for the diagnosis of death on neurological grounds. There is published evidence[28][29][30] strongly suggestive of the persistence of brain stem blood pressure control in organ donors.

A small minority of medical practitioners working in the UK have argued that neither requirement of the UK Health Department's Code of Practice basis for the equation of brain stem death with death is satisfied by its current diagnostic protocol[1] and that in terms of its ability to diagnose de facto brain stem death it falls far short.

2.1.5 References

[1] A Code of Practice for the Diagnosis and Confirmation of Death. Academy of Medical Royal Colleges, 70 Wimpole Street, London, 2008

[2] Criteria for the diagnosis of brain stem death. J Roy Coll Physns of London 1995;29:381-2

[3] The Transplantation of Human Organs Act, 1994. Act No.42 of 1994. s. 2

[4] Human Tissue Transplant Act 2000. s. 19(1)

[5] Controversies in the determination of death. A White Paper by the President's Council on Bioethics, Washington, DC. p 66

[6] Conference of Medical Royal Colleges and their Faculties in the UK. BMJ 1976;2:1187-8

[7] Conference of Medical Royal Colleges and their Faculties in the UK. BMJ 1979;1:332.

[8] Pallis,C. From Brain Death to Brain Stem Death, BMJ, 285, November 1982

[9] Coimbra CG. Implications of ischemic penumbra for the diagnosis of brain death. Brazilian Journal of Medical and Biological Research 1999;32:1479-87

[10] Coimbra CG. The apnoea test – a bedside lethal 'disaster' to avoid a legal 'disaster' in the operating room. In Finis Vitae – is brain death still life? pp.113-145

[11] Saposnik G et al. Problems associated with the apnea test in the diagnosis of brain death. Neurology India 2004;52:342-45

[12] Yingying S et al. Diagnosis of brain death : confirmatory tests after clinical test. Chin Med J 2014;127:1272-77

[13] Coimbra CG. Are 'brain dead' (or 'brain stem dead') patients neurologically recoverable? In Finis Vitae - 'brain death' is not true death. Eds. De Mattei R, Byrne PA. Life Guardian Foundation, Oregon, Ohio, 2009, pp. 313-378

[14] Pallis C, Harley DH. ABC of brain stem death. BMJ Publishing Group, 1996, p.30

[15] Shewmon DA. 'Brain body' disconnection : implications for the theoretical basis of 'brain death'. In Finis Vitae – is brain death still life? Ed. De Mattei R. Consiglio Nazionale delle Richerche. Rubbettino, 2006, pp. 211-250

[16] Powner DJ, Bernstein IM. Extended somatic support for pregnant women after brain death. Crit Care Med 2003;31:1241-49

[17] Evans DW, Lum LC. Cardiac transplantation. Lancet 1980;1:933-4

[18] Evans DW, Lum LC. Brain death. Lancet 1980;2:1022

[19] Evans DW. The demise of 'brain death' in Britain. In Beyond brain death – the case against brain based criteria for human death. Eds. Potts M, Byrne PA, Nilges RG. Kluwer Academic Publishers, 2006, pp. 139-158

[20] G, Magoun HW. Brain stem reticular formation and activation of the EEG. Electroencephalog Clin neurophysiol 1949;1:455-73

[21] Ward AA. The relationship between the bulbar-reticular suppressor region and the EEG. Clin Neurophysiol 1949;1:120

[22] Lindsley DB et al. Effect upon the EEG of acute injury to the brain stem activating system. EEG Clin Neurophysiol 1949;1:475-8627

[23] Parvizi J, Damasio AR. Neuroanatomical correlates of brainstem coma. Brain 2003;126:1524-36

[24] Textbook of clinical neurology, 2nd Edn. Ed. Goetz CG. Elsevier Science, 2003

[25] Bleck TP. In Textbook of clinical neurology, 3rd Edn. Ed. Goetz CG. Elsevier Science, 2007

[26] Zwarts MJ, Kornips FHM. Clinical brainstem death with preserved electroencephalographic activity and visual evoked response. Arch Neurol 2001;58:1010

[27] Tononi G. An information integration theory of consciousness. BMC Neuroscience 2004;5:42

[28] Hall GM et al. Hypothalamic-pituitary function in the 'brain dead' patient. Lancet 1980;2:1259

[29] Wetzel RC et al. Hemodynamic responses in brain dead organ donor patients. Anesthesia and Analgesia 1985;64:125-8

[30] Pennefather SH, Dark JH, Bullock RE. Haemodynamic responses to surgery in brain-dead organ donors. Anaesthesia 1993;48:1034-38

2.1.6 External links

- Great Ormond Street Hospital for Children

2.2 Caloric reflex test

"Nystagmus test" redirects here. For the field sobriety test, see horizontal gaze nystagmus test.

In medicine, the **caloric reflex test** (sometimes termed 'vestibular caloric stimulation') is a test of the vestibulo-ocular reflex that involves irrigating cold or warm water or air into the external auditory canal.

2.2.1 Utility

It is commonly used by physicians, audiologists and other trained professionals to validate a diagnosis of asymmetric function in the peripheral vestibular system. Calorics are usually a subtest of the electronystagmography (ENG) battery of tests. It is one of several tests which can be used to test for brain stem death.

One novel use of this test has been to provide temporary pain relief from phantom limb pains in amputees[1] and paraplegics.[2] It can also induce a temporary remission of anosognosia, the visual and personal aspects of hemispatial neglect, hemianesthesia, and other consequences of right hemispheric damage.[3]

2.2.2 Technique and results

Ice cold or warm water or air is irrigated into the external auditory canal, usually using a syringe. The temperature difference between the body and the injected water creates a convective current in the endolymph of the nearby horizontal semicircular canal. Hot and cold water produce currents in opposite directions and therefore a horizontal nystagmus in opposite directions.[4] In patients with an intact brainstem:

- If the water is warm (44°C or above) endolymph in the ipsilateral horizontal canal rises, causing an increased rate of firing in the vestibular afferent nerve. This situation mimics a head turn to the ipsilateral side. Both eyes will turn toward the contralateral ear, with horizontal nystagmus (quick horizontal eye movements) to the ipsilateral ear.

- If the water is cold, relative to body temperature (30°C or below), the endolymph falls within the semicircular canal, decreasing the rate of vestibular afferent firing. The eyes then turn toward the ipsilateral ear, with horizontal nystagmus to the contralateral ear.[5][6]

Absent reactive eye movement suggests vestibular weakness of the horizontal semicircular canal of the side being stimulated.

In comatose patients with cerebral damage, the fast phase of nystagmus will be absent as this is controlled by the cerebrum. As a result, using cold water irrigation will result in deviation of the eyes toward the ear being irrigated. If both phases are absent, this suggests the patient's brainstem reflexes are also damaged and carries a very poor prognosis.[7]

2.2.3 Mnemonic

One mnemonic used to remember the FAST direction of nystagmus is *COWS*.[8]

COWS: *C*old *O*pposite, *W*arm *S*ame.
Cold water = FAST phase of **nystagmus** to the side
Opposite from the cold water filled ear
Warm water = FAST phase of nystagmus to the **S**ame side as the warm water filled ear
In other words: *Contralateral* when *cold* is applied and *ipsilateral* when *warm* is applied

2.2.4 See also

- Balance disorder

- Inner ear

2.2.5 References

[1] André JM, Martinet N, Paysant J, Beis JM, Le Chapelain L (2001). "Temporary phantom limbs evoked by vestibular caloric stimulation in amputees". *Neuropsychiatry Neuropsychol Behav Neurol* **14** (3): 190–6. PMID 11513103.

[2] Le Chapelain L, Beis JM, Paysant J, André JM (February 2001). "Vestibular caloric stimulation evokes phantom limb illusions in patients with paraplegia". *Spinal Cord* **39** (2): 85–7. doi:10.1038/sj.sc.3101093. PMID 11402363.

[3] Robertson, Ian H.; Marshall, John C. (1993). *Unilateral neglect: clinical and experimental studies*. pp. 111–113. ISBN 978-0-86377-208-5. Retrieved 2010-06-04.

[4] Purves, D; et al. (2004). *Neuroscience*. Sinauer.

[5] *Nystagmus, Acquired* at eMedicine

[6] Narenthiran G. Neurosurgery Quiz.   Annals of Neurosurgery. Accessed on: August 17, 2006.

[7] Mueller-Jensen A, Neunzig HP, Emskötter T (April 1987). "Outcome prediction in comatose patients: significance of reflex eye movement analysis". *J. Neurol. Neurosurg. Psychiatr.* **50** (4): 389–92. doi:10.1136/jnnp.50.4.389. PMC 1031870. PMID 3585347.

[8] Webb C (1985). "COWS caloric test". *Ann Emerg Med* **14** (9): 938. doi:10.1016/S0196-0644(85)80671-5. PMID 4026002.

2.3 Clinical death

Clinical death is the medical term for cessation of blood circulation and breathing, the two necessary criteria to sustain human and many other organisms' lives.[1] It occurs when the heart stops beating in a regular rhythm, a condition called cardiac arrest. The term is also sometimes used in resuscitation research.

Stopped blood circulation has historically proven irreversible in most cases.   Prior to the invention of cardiopulmonary resuscitation (CPR), defibrillation, epinephrine injection, and other treatments in the 20th century, the absence of blood circulation (and vital functions related to blood circulation) was historically considered the official definition of death. With the advent of these strategies, cardiac arrest came to be called *clinical death* rather than simply *death*, to reflect the possibility of post-arrest resuscitation. For medical purposes, it is considered the final physical state before legal death.

At the onset of clinical death, consciousness is lost within several seconds. Measurable brain activity stops within 20 to 40 seconds.[2] Irregular gasping may occur during this early time period, and is sometimes mistaken by rescuers as a sign that CPR is not necessary.[3] During clinical death, all tissues and organs in the body steadily accumulate a type of injury called ischemic injury.

2.3.1 Limits of reversal

Most tissues and organs of the body can survive clinical death for considerable periods. Blood circulation can be stopped in the entire body below the heart for at least 30 minutes, with injury to the spinal cord being a limiting factor.[4] Detached limbs may be successfully reattached after 6 hours of no blood circulation at warm temperatures. Bone, tendon, and skin can survive as long as 8 to 12 hours.[5]

The brain, however, appears to accumulate ischemic injury faster than any other organ. Without special treatment after circulation is restarted, full recovery of the brain after more than 3 minutes of clinical death at normal body temperature is rare.[6][7] Usually brain damage or later brain death results after longer intervals of clinical death even if the heart is restarted and blood circulation is successfully restored. Brain injury is therefore the chief limiting factor for recovery from clinical death.

Although loss of function is almost immediate, there is no specific duration of clinical death at which the non-functioning brain clearly dies. The most vulnerable cells in the brain, CA1 neurons of the hippocampus, are fatally injured by as little as 10 minutes without oxygen. However, the injured cells do not actually die until hours after resuscitation.[8] This delayed death can be prevented *in vitro* by a simple drug treatment even after 20 minutes without oxygen.[9] In other areas of the brain, viable human neurons have been recovered and grown in culture hours after clinical death.[10] Brain failure after clinical death is now known to be due to a complex series of processes called reperfusion injury that occur *after* blood circulation has been restored, especially processes that interfere with blood circulation during the recovery period.[11] Control of these processes is the subject of ongoing research.

In 1990, the laboratory of resuscitation pioneer Peter Safar discovered that reducing body temperature by three degrees Celsius after restarting blood circulation could double the time window of recovery from clinical death without brain damage from 5 minutes to 10 minutes. This induced hypothermia technique is beginning to be used in emergency medicine.[12][13] The combination of mildly reducing body temperature, reducing blood cell concentration, and increasing blood pressure after resuscitation was found especially effective—allowing for recovery of dogs after 12 minutes of clinical death at normal body temperature with practically no brain injury.[14][15] The addition of a drug treatment protocol has been reported to allow recovery of dogs after 16 minutes of clinical death at normal body temperature with no lasting brain injury.[16] Cooling treatment alone has permitted recovery after 17 minutes of clinical death at normal temperature, but with brain injury.[17]

Under laboratory conditions at normal body temperature, the longest period of clinical death of a cat (after complete circulatory arrest) survived with eventual return of brain function is one hour.[18][19]

2.3.2 Hypothermia during clinical death

Reduced body temperature, or therapeutic hypothermia, during clinical death slows the rate of injury accumulation, and extends the time period during which clinical death can be survived. The decrease in the rate of injury can be approximated by the Q_{10} rule, which states that the rate of biochemical reactions decreases by a factor of two for every 10 °C reduction in temperature. As a result, humans can sometimes survive periods of clinical death exceeding one hour at temperatures below 20 °C.[20] The prognosis is improved if clinical death is caused by hypothermia rather than occurring prior to it; in 1999, 29-year-old Swedish woman Anna Bågenholm spent 80 minutes trapped in ice and survived with full recovery from a 13.7 °C core body temperature. It is said in emergency medicine that "nobody is dead until they are warm and dead."[21] In animal studies, up to three hours of clinical death can be survived at temperatures near 0 °C.[22][23]

2.3.3 Life support during clinical death

The purpose of cardiopulmonary resuscitation (CPR) during cardiac arrest is ideally reversal of the clinically dead state by restoration of blood circulation and breathing. However, there is great variation in the effectiveness of CPR for this purpose. Blood pressure is very low during manual CPR,[24] resulting in only a ten-minute average extension of survival.[25] Yet there are cases of patients regaining consciousness during CPR while still in full cardiac arrest.[26] In absence of cerebral function monitoring or frank return to consciousness, the neurological status of patients undergoing CPR is intrinsically uncertain. It is somewhere between the state of clinical death and a normal functioning state.

Patients supported by methods that certainly maintain enough blood circulation and oxygenation for sustaining life during stopped heartbeat and breathing, such as cardiopulmonary bypass, are not customarily considered clinically dead. All parts of the body except the heart and lungs continue to function normally. Clinical death occurs only if machines providing sole circulatory support are turned off.

2.3.4   Controlled clinical death

Certain surgeries for cerebral aneurysms or aortic arch defects require that blood circulation be stopped while repairs are performed. This deliberate temporary induction of clinical death is called circulatory arrest. It is typically performed by lowering body temperature between 18 °C (64 °F) and 20 °C (68 °F) and stopping the heart and lungs. This state is called deep hypothermic circulatory arrest. At such low temperatures most patients can tolerate the clinically dead state for up to 30 minutes without incurring significant brain injury.[27] Longer durations are possible at lower temperatures, but the usefulness of longer procedures has not been established yet.[28]

Controlled clinical death has also been proposed as a treatment for exsanguinating trauma to create time for surgical repair.[29]

2.3.5   Clinical death and the determination of death

Main article: Medical definition of death

Death was historically believed to be an event that coincided with the onset of clinical death. It is now understood that death is a series of physical events, not a single one, and determination of permanent death is dependent on other factors beyond simple cessation of breathing and heartbeat.[11]

Clinical death that occurs unexpectedly is treated as a medical emergency. CPR is initiated. In a United States hospital, a Code Blue is declared and Advanced Cardiac Life Support procedures used to attempt to restart a normal heartbeat. This effort continues until either the heart is restarted, or a physician determines that continued efforts are useless and recovery is impossible. If this determination is made, the physician pronounces legal death and resuscitation efforts stop.

If clinical death is expected due to terminal illness or withdrawal of supportive care, often a Do Not Resuscitate (DNR) or "no code" order is in place. This means that no resuscitation efforts are made, and a physician or nurse may pronounce legal death at the onset of clinical death.

A patient with working heart and lungs who is determined to be brain dead can be pronounced legally dead without clinical death occurring. However, some courts have been reluctant to impose such a determination over the religious objections of family members, such as in the Jesse Koochin case.[30] Similar issues were also raised by the case of Mordechai Dov Brody, but the child died before a court could resolve the matter.[31] Conversely, in the case of Marlise Muñoz, a hospital refused to remove a brain

dead woman from life support machines for nearly two months, despite her husband's requests, because she was pregnant.[32]

2.3.6   See also

- Death
- Brain death
- Legal death
- Cardiac arrest
- Therapeutic hypothermia
- Information-theoretic death
- Lazarus phenomenon
- Near-death experience

2.3.7   References

[1] Kastenbaum, Robert (2006). "Definitions of Death". *Encyclopedia of Death and Dying*. Retrieved 27 January 2007.

[2] Lind B, B; Snyder, J; Kampschulte, S; Safar, P; et al. (1975). "A review of total brain ischaemia models in dogs and original experiments on clamping the aorta". *Resuscitation* (Elsevier) **4** (1): 19–31. doi:10.1016/0300-9572(75)90061-1. PMID 1188189.

[3] Eisenberg MS, MS (2006). "Incidence and significance of gasping or agonal respirations in cardiac arrest patients". *Current Opinion in Critical Care* (Elsevier) **12** (3): 189–192. doi:10.1097/01.ccx.0000224862.48087.66. PMID 16672777.

[4] Hazim J, HJ; Winnerkvist, A; Miller Cc, 3rd; Iliopoulos, DC; Reardon, MJ; Espada, R; Baldwin, JC (1998). "Effect of extended cross-clamp time during thoracoabdominal aortic aneurysm repair". *The Annals of Thoracic Surgery* (The Society of Thoracic Surgeons) **66** (4): 1204–8. doi:10.1016/S0003-4975(98)00781-4. PMID 9800807.

[5] *Replantation* at eMedicine

[6] Safar P, P (1986). "Cerebral resuscitation after cardiac arrest: a review". *Circulation* (Lippincott Williams & Wilkins) **74** (6 Pt 2): IV138–153. PMID 3536160.

[7] Safar P, P (1988). "Resuscitation from clinical death: pathophysiologic limits and therapeutic potentials". *Critical Care Medicine* (Lippincott Williams & Wilkins) **16** (10): 923–41. doi:10.1097/00003246-198810000-00003. PMID 3048894.

[8] Kirino T, T (2000). "Delayed neuronal death". *Neuropathology* **20**: S95–7. doi:10.1046/j.1440-1789.2000.00306.x. PMID 11037198.

[9] Popovic R, R; Liniger, R; Bickler, PE (2000). "Anesthetics and mild hypothermia similarly prevent hippocampal neuron death in an in vitro model of cerebral ischemia". *Anesthesiology* (Lippincott Williams & Wilkins) **92** (5): 1343–9. doi:10.1097/00000542-200005000-00024. PMID 10781280.

[10] Kim SU, SU; Warren, KG; Kalia, M; et al. (1979). "Tissue culture of adult human neurons". *Neuroscience Letters* (Elsevier Scientific Publishers Ireland) **11** (2): 137–141. doi:10.1016/0304-3940(79)90116-2. PMID 313541.

[11] Crippen, David. "Brain Failure and Brain Death: Introduction". *ACS Surgery Online, Critical Care, April 2005.* Archived from the original on 11 October 2007. Retrieved 9 January 2007.

[12] Holzer M, Behringer W, M; Behringer, W (2005). "Therapeutic hypothermia after cardiac arrest". *Current Opinion in Anesthesiology* (Lippincott Williams & Wilkins) **18** (2): 163–8. doi:10.1097/01.aco.0000162835.33474.a9. PMID 16534333.

[13] Davis, Robert (11 December 2006). "To treat cardiac arrest, doctors cool the body". USA Today. Retrieved 7 January 2007.

[14] Leonov Y, Y; Sterz, F; Safar, P; Radovsky, A; Oku, K; Tisherman, S; Stezoski, SW; et al. (1990). "Mild cerebral hypothermia during and after cardiac arrest improves neurologic outcome in dogs". *Journal of cerebral blood flow and metabolism* (Nature Pub. Group) **10** (1): 57–70. doi:10.1038/jcbfm.1990.8. PMID 2298837.

[15] Safar P, P; Xiao, F; Radovsky, A; Tanigawa, K; Ebmeyer, U; Bircher, N; Alexander, H; Stezoski, SW; et al. (1996). "Improved cerebral resuscitation from cardiac arrest in dogs with mild hypothermia plus blood flow promotion". *Stroke* (Lippincott Williams & Wilkins) **27** (1): 105–113. doi:10.1161/01.STR.27.1.105. PMID 8553385.

[16] Lemler J, J; Harris, SB; Platt, C; Huffman, TM; et al. (2004). "The arrest of biological time as a bridge to engineered negligible senescence". *Annals of the New York Academy of Sciences* (New York Academy of Sciences) **1019**: 559–63. doi:10.1196/annals.1297.104. PMID 15247086.

[17] Leonov Y, Y; Sterz, F; Safar, P; Radovsky, A; et al. (1990). "Moderate hypothermia after cardiac arrest of 17 minutes in dogs. Effect on cerebral and cardiac outcome". *Stroke* (Lippincott Williams & Wilkins) **21** (11): 1600–6. doi:10.1161/01.STR.21.11.1600. PMID 2237954.

[18] Hossmann KA, KA; Sato, K; et al. (1970). "Recovery of Neuronal Function after Prolonged Cerebral Ischemia". *Science* (American Association for the Advancement of Science) **168** (3929): 375–6. doi:10.1126/science.168.3929.375. PMID 4908037.

[19] Hossmann KA, KA; Schmidt-Kastner, R; Grosse Ophoff, B; et al. (1987). "Recovery of integrative central nervous function after one hour global cerebro-circulatory arrest in normothermic cat". *Journal of the Neurological Sciences* (Elsevier) **77** (2–3): 305–20. doi:10.1016/0022-510X(87)90130-4. PMID 3819770.

[20] Walpoth BH, BH; Locher, T; Leupi, F; Schüpbach, P; Mühlemann, W; Althaus, U; et al. (1990). "Accidental deep hypothermia with cardiopulmonary arrest: extracorporeal blood rewarming in 11 patients". *European Journal of Cardio-Thoracic Surgery* (Elsevier Science) **4** (7): 390–3. doi:10.1016/1010-7940(90)90048-5. PMID 2397132.

[21] "Skier revived from clinical death". *BBC News.* 18 January 2000. Retrieved 9 January 2007.

[22] Haneda K, K; Thomas, R; Sands, MP; Breazeale, DG; Dillard, DH; et al. (1986). "Whole body protection during three hours of total circulatory arrest: an experimental study". *Cryobiology* (Academic Press) **23** (6): 483–94. doi:10.1016/0011-2240(86)90057-X. PMID 3802887.

[23] Behringer W, Safar P, W; Safar, P; Wu, X; Kentner, R; Radovsky, A; Kochanek, PM; Dixon, CE; Tisherman, SA; et al. (2003). "Survival without brain damage after clinical death of 60–120 mins in dogs using suspended animation by profound hypothermia". *Critical Care Medicine* (Lippincott Williams & Wilkins) **31** (5): 1592–3. doi:10.1097/01.CCM.0000063450.73967.40. PMID 12771628.

[24] Chandra NC, NC; Tsitlik, JE; Halperin, HR; Guerci, AD; Weisfeldt, ML; et al. (1990). "Observations of hemodynamics during human cardiopulmonary resuscitation". *Critical Care Medicine* (Lippincott Williams & Wilkins) **18** (9): 929–34. doi:10.1097/00003246-199009000-00005. PMID 2394116.

[25] Cummins RO, RO; Eisenberg, MS; Hallstrom, AP; Litwin, PE; et al. (1985). "Survival of out-of-hospital cardiac arrest with early initiation of cardiopulmonary resuscitation". *The American Journal of Emergency Medicine* (W B Saunders) **3** (2): 114–9. doi:10.1016/0735-6757(85)90032-4. PMID 3970766,

[26] Lewinter JR, JR; Carden, DL; Nowak, RM; Enriquez, E; Martin, GB; et al. (1989). "CPR-dependent consciousness: evidence for cardiac compression causing forward flow". *Annals of Emergency Medicine* (Mosby) **18** (10): 1111–5. doi:10.1016/S0196-0644(89)80942-4. PMID 2802288.

[27] Conolly, S; Arrowsmith, JE; Klein, AA (2010). "Deep hypothermic circulatory arrest". *Continuing Education in Anaesthesia, Critical Care & Pain* **10** (5): 138–142. doi:10.1093/bjaceaccp/mkq024.

[28] Greenberg, Mark S (15 February 2010). *Handbook of Neurosurgery.* Thieme. p. 1063. ISBN 978-1-60406-326-4. Retrieved 18 November 2012.

[29] Bellamy, R.; Safar, P.; Tisherman, S. A.; Basford, R.; Brut-
      tig, S. P.; Capone, A.; Dubick, M. A.; Ernster, L.; Hattler Jr,
      B. G.; Hochachka, P.; Klain, M.; Kochanek, P. M.; Kofke,
      W. A.; Lancaster, J. R.; McGowan Jr, F. X.; Oeltgen, P. R.;
      Severinghaus, J. W.; Taylor, M. J.; Zar, H. (1996). "Sus-
      pended animation for delayed resuscitation". *Critical care
      medicine* **24** (2 Suppl): S24–S47. PMID 8608704.

[30] Appel, JM. Defining Death: When Physicians and Families
      Differ" *Journal of Medical Ethics* Fall 2005

[31] "Brain-dead NYC boy at center of care controversy dies -
      USATODAY.com". usatoday.com.   16 November 2008.
      Retrieved November 17, 2008.

[32] "Texas judge: Remove brain-dead woman from ventilator,
      other machines". CNN. January 24, 2014.

2.4   Coma

For other uses, see Coma (disambiguation) and Comas
(disambiguation).
Not to be confused with Comma.

In medicine, **coma** (from the Greek κῶμα *koma*, meaning "deep sleep")[1] is a state of unconsciousness in which
a person: cannot be awakened; fails to respond normally to
painful stimuli, light, or sound; lacks a normal wake-sleep
cycle; and does not initiate voluntary actions.[2] A person in
a state of coma is described as being **comatose**. Typically,
a distinction is made in the medical community between a
coma and a medically induced coma, the former is generally
understood to be a result of circumstances beyond the control of the medical community, while the latter is generally
understood to be a means by which medical professionals
may allow a patient's injuries to heal in a controlled environment.

A comatose person exhibits a complete absence of wakefulness and is unable to consciously feel, speak, hear, or
move.[3] For a patient to maintain consciousness, two important neurological components must function. The first
is the cerebral cortex—the gray matter that forms the outer
layer of the brain. The other is a structure located in the
brainstem, called reticular activating system (RAS).[4][5] Injury to either or both of these components is sufficient to
cause a patient to experience a coma. The cerebral cortex is a group of tight, dense, "gray matter" composed of
the nuclei of the neurons whose axons then form the "white
matter", and is responsible for perception, relay of the sensory input (sensation) via the thalamic pathway, and many
other neurological functions, including complex thinking.

RAS, on the other hand, is a more primitive structure in the
brainstem that is tightly in connection with reticular formation (RF). The RAS area of the brain has two tracts,

the ascending and descending tract. Made up of a system
of acetylcholine-producing neurons, the ascending track,
or ascending reticular activating system (ARAS), works to
arouse and wake up the brain, from the RF, through the thalamus, and then finally to the cerebral cortex.[6] A failure in
ARAS functioning may then lead to a coma.

2.4.1   Signs and symptoms

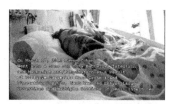

Image of a man in a coma.[7]

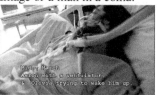

Image of the man still unresponsive to stimuli.[8]

Generally, a person who is unable to voluntarily open the
eyes, does not have a sleep-wake cycle, is unresponsive in
spite of strong tactile (painful), or verbal stimuli and who
generally scores between 3 to 8[9] on the Glasgow Coma
Scale is considered in a coma.[2] Coma may have developed
in humans as a response to injury to allow the body to pause
bodily actions and heal the most immediate injuries - if at
all - before waking. It therefore could be a compensatory
state in which the body's expenditure of energy is not su-
perfluous. The severity and mode of onset of coma depends
on the underlying cause. For instance, severe hypoglycemia
(low blood sugar) or hypercapnia (increased carbon dioxide
levels in the blood) initially cause mild agitation and confusion, but progress to obtundation, stupor and finally complete unconsciousness. In contrast, coma resulting from a
severe traumatic brain injury or subarachnoid hemorrhage
can be instantaneous. The mode of onset may therefore be
indicative of the underlying cause.

Causes of coma

Coma may result from a variety of conditions, including intoxication (such as drug abuse, overdose or mis-
use of over the counter medications, prescribed medication, or controlled substances), metabolic abnormalities, central nervous system diseases, acute neurologic injuries such as strokes or herniations, hypoxia, hypothermia,
hypoglycemia, Eclampsia or traumatic injuries such as head

trauma caused by falls or vehicle collisions. It may also be deliberately induced by pharmaceutical agents during major neurosurgery, to preserve higher brain functions following brain trauma, or to save the patient from extreme pain during healing of injuries or diseases.[10]

Forty percent of comatose states result from drug poisoning.[11] Drugs damage or weaken the synaptic functioning in the ARAS and keep the system from properly functioning to arouse the brain.[6] Secondary effects of drugs, which include abnormal heart rate and blood pressure, as well as abnormal breathing and sweating, may also indirectly harm the functioning of the ARAS and lead to a coma. Seizures and hallucinations have shown to also play a major role in ARAS malfunction. Given that drug poisoning is the cause for a large portion of patients in a coma, hospitals first test all comatose patients by observing pupil size and eye movement, through the vestibular-ocular reflex.[6]

The second most common cause of coma, which makes up about 25% of comatose patients, occurs from lack of oxygen, generally resulting from cardiac arrest.[11] The Central Nervous System (CNS) requires a great deal of oxygen for its neurons. Oxygen deprivation in the brain, also known as hypoxia, causes neuronal extracellular sodium and calcium to decrease and intracellular calcium to increase, which harms neuron communication.[12] Lack of oxygen in the brain also causes ATP exhaustion and cellular breakdown from cytoskeleton damage and nitric oxide production.

Twenty percent of comatose states result from the side effects of a stroke.[11] During a stroke, blood flow to part of the brain is restricted or blocked. An ischemic stroke, brain hemorrhage, or tumor may cause such cessation of blood flow. Lack of blood to cells in the brain prevents oxygen from getting to the neurons, and consequently causes cells to become disrupted and eventually die. As brain cells die, brain tissue continues to deteriorate, which may affect functioning of the ARAS.

The remaining 15% of comatose cases result from trauma, excessive blood loss, malnutrition, hypothermia, hyperthermia, abnormal glucose levels, and many other biological disorders.

2.4.2 Diagnosis

Diagnosis of coma is simple, but diagnosing the cause of the underlying disease process is often challenging. The first priority in treatment of a comatose patient is stabilization following the basic ABCs (standing for airway, breathing, and circulation). Once a person in a coma is stable, investigations are performed to assess the underlying cause. Investigative methods are divided into physical examination findings and imaging (such as CAT scan, MRI, etc.) and special studies (EEG, etc.)

Diagnostic steps

When an unconscious patient enters a hospital, the hospital utilizes a series of diagnostic steps to identify the cause of unconsciousness. According to Young,[6] the following steps should be taken when dealing with a patient possibly in a coma:

1. Perform a general examination and medical history check

2. Make sure the patient is in an actual comatose state and or is not in locked-in state (patient is either able to voluntarily move his eyes or blink) or psychogenic unresponsiveness (caloric stimulation of the vestibular apparatus results in slow deviation of eyes towards the stimulation followed by rapid correction to mid-line. This response cannot be voluntarily suppressed, so if the patient does not have this response, psychogenic coma can be ruled out.)

3. Find the site of the brain that may be causing coma (i.e., brain stem, back of brain...) and assess the severity of the coma with the Glasgow coma scale

4. Take blood work to see if drugs were involved or if it was a result of hypoventilation/hyperventilation

5. Check for levels of "serum glucose, calcium, sodium, potassium, magnesium, phosphate, urea, and creatinine"

6. Perform brain scans to observe any abnormal brain functioning using either CT or MRI scans

7. Continue to monitor brain waves and identify seizures of patient using EEGs

Initial assessment and evaluation

In the initial assessment of coma, it is common to gauge the level of consciousness by spontaneously exhibited actions, response to vocal stimuli ("Can you hear me?"), and painful stimuli; this is known as the AVPU (alert, vocal stimuli, painful stimuli, unresponsive) scale. More elaborate scales, such as the Glasgow Coma Scale, quantify an individual's reactions such as eye opening, movement and verbal response on a scale; Glasgow Coma Scale (GCS) is an indication of the extent of brain injury varying from 3 (indicating severe brain injury and death) to a maximum of 15 (indicating mild or no brain injury).

In those with deep unconsciousness, there is a risk of asphyxiation as the control over the muscles in the face and throat is diminished. As a result, those presenting to a hospital with coma are typically assessed for this risk ("airway management"). If the risk of asphyxiation is deemed high, doctors may use various devices (such as an oropharyngeal airway, nasopharyngeal airway or endotracheal tube) to safeguard the airway.

Physical examination findings

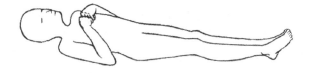

Decorticate posturing, indicating a lesion at the red nucleus or above. This positioning is stereotypical for upper brain stem, or cortical damage. The other variant is decerebrate posturing, not seen in this picture.

Physical examination is critical after stabilization. It should include vital signs, a general portion dedicated to making observations about the patient's respiration (breathing pattern), body movements (if any), and of the patient's body habitus (physique); it should also include assessment of the brainstem and cortical function through special reflex tests such as the oculocephalic reflex test (doll's eyes test), oculovestibular reflex test (cold caloric test), nasal tickle, corneal reflex, and the gag reflex.

Vital signs in medicine are temperature (rectal is most accurate), blood pressure, heart rate (pulse), respiratory rate, and oxygen saturation. It should be easy to evaluate these vitals quickly to gain insight into a patient's metabolism, fluid status, heart function, vascular integrity, and tissue oxygenation.

Respiratory pattern (breathing rhythm) is significant and should be noted in a comatose patient. Certain stereotypical patterns of breathing have been identified including Cheyne–Stokes, a form of breathing in which the patient's breathing pattern is described as alternating episodes of hyperventilation and apnea. This is a dangerous pattern and is often seen in pending herniations, extensive cortical lesions, or brainstem damage.[4] Another pattern of breathing is apneustic breathing, which is characterized by sudden pauses of inspiration and is due to a lesion of the pons.[2][4] Ataxic breathing is irregular and is due to a lesion (damage) of the medulla.

Assessment of posture and body habitus is the next step. It involves general observation about the patient's positioning. There are often two stereotypical postures seen in comatose patients. Decorticate posturing is a stereotypical posturing in which the patient has arms flexed at the elbow, and arms adducted toward the body, with both legs extended.

Decerebrate posturing is a stereotypical posturing in which the legs are similarly extended (stretched), but the arms are also stretched (extended at the elbow). The posturing is critical since it indicates where the damage is in the central nervous system. A decorticate posturing indicates a lesion (a point of damage) at or above the red nucleus, whereas a decerebrate posturing indicates a lesion at or below the red nucleus. In other words, a decorticate lesion is closer to the cortex, as opposed to a decerebrate cortex that is closer to the brainstem.

Oculocephalic reflex also known as the doll's eye is performed to assess the integrity of the brainstem. Patient's eyelids are gently elevated and the cornea is visualized. The patient's head is then moved to the patient's left, to observe if the eyes stay or deviate toward the patient's right; same maneuver is attempted on the opposite side. If the patient's eyes move in a direction opposite to the direction of the rotation of the head, then the patient is said to have an intact brainstem. However, failure of both eyes to move to one side, can indicate damage or destruction of the affected side. In special cases, where only one eye deviates and the other does not, this often indicates a lesion (or damage) of the medial longitudinal fasciculus (MLF), which is a brainstem nerve tract. Caloric reflex test also evaluates both cortical and brainstem function; cold water is injected into one ear and the patient is observed for eye movement; if the patient's eyes slowly deviate toward the ear where the water was injected, then the brainstem is intact, however failure to deviate toward the injected ear indicates damage of the brainstem on that side. Cortex is responsible for a rapid nystagmus away from this deviated position and is often seen in patients who are conscious or merely lethargic.

An important part of the physical exam is also assessment of the cranial nerves. Due to the unconscious status of the patient, only a limited number of the nerves can be assessed. These include the cranial nerves number 2 (CN II), number 3 (CN III), number 5 (CN V), number 7 (CN VII), and cranial nerves 9 and 10 (CN IX, CN X). Gag reflex helps assess cranial nerves 9 and 10. Pupil reaction to light is important because it shows an intact retina, and cranial nerve number 2 (CN II); if pupils are reactive to light, then that also indicates that the cranial nerve number 3 (CN III) (or at least its parasympathetic fibers) are intact. Corneal reflex assess the integrity of cranial nerve number 7 (CN VII), and cranial nerve number 5 (CN V). Cranial nerve number 5 (CN V), and its ophthalmic branch (V_1) are responsible for the afferent arm of the reflex, and the cranial nerve number 7 (CN VII) also known a facial nerve, is responsible for the efferent arm, causing contraction of the muscle orbicularis oculi resulting in closing of the eyes.

Pupil assessment is often a critical portion of a comatose examination, as it can give information as to the cause of the coma; the following table is a technical, medical guideline for common pupil findings and their possible interpretations:[4]

Imaging and special tests findings

Imaging basically encompasses computed tomography (CAT or CT) scan of the brain, or MRI for example, and is performed to identify specific causes of the coma, such as hemorrhage in the brain or herniation of the brain structures. Special tests such as an EEG can also show a lot about the activity level of the cortex such as semantic processing,[13] presence of seizures, and are important available tools not only for the assessment of the cortical activity but also for predicting the likelihood of the patient's awakening.[14] The autonomous responses such as the skin conductance response may also provide further insight on the patient's emotional processing.[15]

History

When diagnosing any neurological condition, history and examination are fundamental. History is obtained by family, friends or EMS. The Glasgow Coma Scale is a helpful system used to examine and determine the depth of coma, track patients progress and predict outcome as best as possible. In general a correct diagnosis can be achieved by combining findings from physical exam, imaging, and history components and directs the appropriate therapy.

Severity and classification

Main article: Coma scale

A coma can be classified as (1) supratentoral (above Tentorium cerebelli), (2) infratentoral (below Tentorium cerebelli), (3) metabolic or (4) diffused.[4] This classification is merely dependent on the position of the original damage that caused the coma, and does not correlate with severity or the prognosis. The severity of coma impairment however is categorized into several levels. Patients may or may not progress through these levels. In the first level, the brain responsiveness lessens, normal reflexes are lost, the patient no longer responds to pain and cannot hear.

The Rancho Los Amigos Scale is a complex scale that has eight separate levels, and is often used in the first few weeks or months of coma while the patient is under closer observation, and when shifts between levels are more frequent.

2.4.3   Treatment

Medical treatment

The treatment hospitals use on comatose patients depends on both the severity and cause of the comatose state. Although the best treatment for comatose patients remains unknown, hospitals usually place comatose patients in an Intensive Care Unit (ICU) immediately.[6] In the ICU, the hospital monitors a patient's breathing and brain activity through CT scans. Attention must first be directed to maintaining the patient's respiration and circulation, using intubation and ventilation, administration of intravenous fluids or blood and other supportive care as needed. Once a patient is stable and no longer in immediate danger, the medical staff may concentrate on maintaining the health of patient's physical state. The concentration is directed to preventing infections such as pneumonias, bedsores (decubitus ulcers), and providing balanced nutrition.[16] These infections may appear from the patient not being able to move around, and being confined to the bed. The nursing staff moves the patient every 2–3 hours from side to side and depending on the state of consciousness sometimes to a chair. The goal is to move the patient as much as possible to try to avoid bedsores, atelectasis and pneumonia. Pneumonia can occur from the person's inability to swallow leading to aspiration, lack of gag reflex or from feeding tube, (aspiration pneumonia). Physical therapy may also be used to prevent contractures and orthopedic deformities that would limit recovery for those patients who emerge from coma.

A person in a coma may become restless, or seize and need special care to prevent them from hurting themselves. Medicine may be given to calm such individuals. Patients who are restless may also try to pull on tubes or dressings so soft cloth wrist restraints may be put on. Side rails on the bed should be kept up to prevent the patient from falling.[16]

In attempt to wake comatose patients, some hospitals treat their patients by either reversing the cause of comatose (i.e., glucose shock if low sugar), giving medication to stop brain swelling, or inducing hypothermia. Inducing hypothermia on comatose patients provides one of the main treatments for patients after suffering from cardiac arrest. In this treatment, medical personnel expose patients to "external or intravascular cooling" at 32-34 °C for 24 h.; this treatment cools patients down about 2-3 °C less than normal body temperature.[17] In 2002, Baldursdottir and her coworkers[17] found that in the hospital, more comatose patients survived after induced hypothermia than patients that remained at normal body temperature. For this reason, the hospital chose to continue the induced hypothermia technique for all of its comatose patients that suffered from cardiac arrest.[17]

Emotional challenges

Coma has a wide variety of emotional reactions from the family members of the affected patients, as well as the primary care givers taking care of the patients. Common reactions, such as desperation, anger, frustration, and denial are possible. The focus of the patient care should be on creating an amicable relationship with the family members or dependents of a comatose patient as well as creating a rapport with the medical staff.[18]

2.4.4 Prognosis

Comas can last from several days to several weeks. In more severe cases a coma may last for over five weeks, while some have lasted as long as several years. After this time, some patients gradually come out of the coma, some progress to a vegetative state, and others die. Some patients who have entered a vegetative state go on to regain a degree of awareness. Others remain in a vegetative state for years or even decades (the longest recorded period being 42 years).[19][20]

The outcome for coma and vegetative state depends on the cause, location, severity and extent of neurological damage. A deeper coma alone does not necessarily mean a slimmer chance of recovery, because some people in deep coma recover well while others in a so-called milder coma sometimes fail to improve.

People may emerge from a coma with a combination of physical, intellectual and psychological difficulties that need special attention. Recovery usually occurs gradually—patients acquire more and more ability to respond. Some patients never progress beyond very basic responses, but many recover full awareness.[21] Regaining consciousness is not instant: in the first days, patients are only awake for a few minutes, and duration of time awake gradually increases. This is unlike the situation in many movies where people who awake from comas are instantly able to continue their normal lives. In reality, the coma patient awakes sometimes in a profound state of confusion, not knowing how they got there and sometimes suffering from dysarthria, the inability to articulate any speech, and with many other disabilities.

Predicted chances of recovery are variable owing to different techniques used to measure the extent of neurological damage. All the predictions are based on statistical rates with some level of chance for recovery present: a person with a low chance of recovery may still awaken. Time is the best general predictor of a chance of recovery: after four months of coma caused by brain damage, the chance of partial recovery is less than 15%, and the chance of full recovery is very low.[22]

The most common cause of death for a person in a vegeta-

tive state is secondary infection such as pneumonia, which can occur in patients who lie still for extended periods.

There are reports of patients coming out of coma after long periods of time. After 19 years in a minimally conscious state, Terry Wallis spontaneously began speaking and regained awareness of his surroundings.[23] Similarly, Polish railroad worker Jan Grzebski woke up from a 19-year coma in 2007.

A brain-damaged man, trapped in a coma-like state for six years, was brought back to consciousness in 2003 by doctors who planted electrodes deep inside his brain. The method, called deep brain stimulation (DBS) successfully roused communication, complex movement and eating ability in the 38-year-old American man who suffered a traumatic brain injury. His injuries left him in a minimally conscious state (MCS), a condition akin to a coma but characterized by occasional, but brief, evidence of environmental and self-awareness that coma patients lack.[24]

Comas lasting seconds to minutes result in post-traumatic amnesia (PTA) that lasts hours to days; recovery plateau occurs over days to weeks. Comas that last hours to days result in PTA lasting days to weeks; recovery plateau occurs over months. Comas lasting weeks result in PTA that lasts months; recovery plateau occurs over months to years.[25]

2.4.5 Society and culture

Research by Dr. Eelco Wijdicks on the depiction of comas in movies was published in Neurology in May 2006. Dr. Wijdicks studied 30 films (made between 1970 and 2004) that portrayed actors in prolonged comas, and he concluded that only two films accurately depicted the state of a coma victim and the agony of waiting for a patient to awaken: *Reversal of Fortune* (1990) and *The Dreamlife of Angels* (1998). The remaining 28 were criticized for portraying miraculous awakenings with no lasting side effects, unrealistic depictions of treatments and equipment required, and comatose patients remaining muscular and tanned.[26]

2.4.6 See also

- Brain death, lack of activity in both cortex, and lack of brainstem function

- Coma scale, a system to assess the severity of coma

- Locked-in syndrome, Paralysis of most muscles, except ocular muscles of the eyes, while patient is conscious

- Persistent vegetative state (vegetative coma), deep coma without detectable awareness. Damage to the cortex, with an intact brainstem.

- Process Oriented Coma Work, for an approach to working with residual consciousness in comatose patients.

2.4.7 References

[1] *"Coma* Origin". Online Etymology Dictionary. Retrieved 14 August 2015.

[2] Weyhenmyeye, James A.; Eve A. Gallman (2007). *Rapid Review Neuroscience 1st Ed.* Mosby Elsevier. pp. 177–9. ISBN 0-323-02261-8.

[3] Bordini, A.L.; Luiz, T.F.; Fernandes, M.; Arruda, W. O.; Teive, H. A. (2010). "Coma scales: a historical review". *Arquivos de neuro-psiquiatria* **68** (6): 930–937. doi:10.1590/S0004-282X2010000600019. PMID 21243255.

[4] Hannaman, Robert A. (2005). *MedStudy Internal Medicine Review Core Curriculum: Neurology 11th Ed.* MedStudy. pp. (11–1) to (11–2). ISBN 1-932703-01-2.

[5] "Persistent vegetative state: A medical minefield". *New Scientist*: 40–3. July 7, 2007. See diagram.

[6] Young, G.B. (2009). "Coma". *Ann N Y Acad . BjjSci* **1157** (1157): 32–47. Bibcode:2009NYASA1157...32Y. doi:10.1111/j.1749-6632.2009.04471.x.

[7] "Video of man at beginning of documented 3 month coma.".

[8] "Video of man still nonresponsive to stimuli while in coma.".

[9] Russ Rowlett. "Glasgow Coma Scale". University of North Carolina at Chapel Hill.

[10] Benjamin Werdro. "Induced Coma".

[11] Liversedge, Timothy; Hirsch (2010). "Coma". *Anaesthesia & Intensive Care Medicine* **11** (9): 337–339. doi:10.1016/j.mpaic.2010.05.008.

[12] Busl, K. M.; Greer, D. M. (2010). "Hypoxic-ischemic brain injury: Pathophysiology, neuropathology and mechanisms". *NeuroRehabilitation*: 5–13.

[13] Daltrozzo, J., Wioland, N., Mutschler, V., Lutun, P., Jaeger, A., Calon, B., Meyer, A., Pottecher, T., Lang, S., Kotchoubey, B. (2009c). Cortical Information Processing in Coma, Cognitive & Behavioral Neurology, 22(1), 53-62.

[14] Daltrozzo, J., Wioland, N., Mutschler, V., Kotchoubey, B. (2007). Predicting Coma and other Low Responsive Patients Outcome using Event-Related Brain Potentials: A Meta-analysis. Clinical Neurophysiology, 118, 606-614.

[15] Daltrozzo, J., Wioland, N., Mutschler, V., Lutun, P., Calon, B., Meyer, A., Jaeger, A., Pottecher, T., Kotchoubey, B. (2010a). Electrodermal Response in Coma and Other Low Responsive Patients. Neuroscience Letters, 475(1), 44-47.

[16] "Coma" (PDF). Retrieved 2010-12-08.

[17] Baldursdottir, S.; Sigvaldason, K.; Karason, S.; Valsson, F.; Sigurdsson, G. H. (2010). "Induced hypothermia in comatose survivors of asphyxia: a case series of 14 consecutive cases". *Acta Anaesthesiol. Scand.* **54** (7): 821–826. doi:10.1111/j.1399-6576.2010.02248.x. PMID 20497127.

[18] Coma Care (2010-03-30). "Caring for Care Giver and Family". Retrieved 2010-12-08.

[19] Edwarda O'Bara, who spent 4 decades in a coma, dies at 59

[20] Aruna Shanba, who spent 42 years in coma.

[21] NINDS (October 29, 2010). "Coma Information Page: National Institute of Neurological Disorders and Stroke (NINDS)". Retrieved 2010-12-08.

[22] Formisano R; Carlesimo GA; Sabbadini M; et al. (May 2004). "Clinical predictors and neuropleropsychological outcome in severe traumatic brain injury patients". *Acta Neurochir (Wien)* **146** (5): 457–62. doi:10.1007/s00701-004-0225-4. PMID 15118882.

[23] "Mother stunned by coma victim's unexpected words". *The Sydney Morning Herald*. 2003-07-12.

[24] "Electrodes stir man from six-year coma-like state". *Cosmos Magazine*. 2 August 2007.

[25] "Post-traumatic amnesia".

[26] Eelco F.M. Wijdicks, MD and Coen A. Wijdicks, BS (2006). "The portrayal of coma in contemporary motion pictures". *Neurology* **66** (9): 1300–1303. doi:10.1212/01.wnl.0000210497.62202.e9. PMID 16682658. Retrieved 2009-11-25.

2.5 Corneal reflex

The **corneal reflex**, also known as the **blink reflex**, is an involuntary blinking of the eyelids elicited by stimulation of the cornea (such as by touching or by a foreign body), or bright light, though could result from any peripheral stimulus. Stimulation should elicit both a direct and consensual response (response of the opposite eye). The reflex occurs at a rapid rate of 0.1s. The purpose of this reflex is to protect the eyes from foreign bodies and bright lights (the latter known as the optical reflex).[1] The blink reflex also occurs when sounds greater than 40-60 dB are made.[2]

The reflex is mediated by:

- the nasociliary branch of the ophthalmic branch (V_1) of the 5th cranial nerve (trigeminal nerve) sensing the stimulus on the cornea, lid, or conjunctiva (i.e. it is the afferent).

- the temporal and zygomatic branches of the 7th cranial nerve (Facial nerve) initiating the motor response (i.e. it is the efferent).

- Mediated by centre in the pons of brainstem.

Use of contact lenses may diminish or abolish the testing of this reflex.

The optical reflex, on the other hand, is slower and is mediated by the visual cortex, which resides in the occipital lobe of the brain. The reflex is absent in infants under 9 months.

The examination of the corneal reflex is a part of some neurological exams, particularly when evaluating coma. Damage to the ophthalmic branch (V_1) of the 5th cranial nerve results in absent corneal reflex when the affected eye is stimulated. Stimulation of one cornea normally has a consensual response, with both eyelids normally closing.

2.5.1   Rates

When awake, the lids spread the tear secretions over the corneal surface, on a typical basis of 2 to 10 seconds (though this may vary individually). However, blinking is not only dependent on dryness and/or irritation. A brain area, the globus pallidus of the basal ganglia, contains a blinking center that controls blinking. Nonetheless, the external stimuli are still involved. Blinking is linked with the extraocular muscles. Blinking is often concurrent with a shift in gaze, and it is believed that this helps the movement of the eye.

2.5.2   See also

- Reflex

- Menace reflex

2.5.3   References

[1] "eye, human."Encyclopædia Britannica from Encyclopædia Britannica 2006 Ultimate Reference Suite DVD 2009

[2] Garde, M.M., & Cowey, A. (2000). *"Deaf hearing": Unacknowledged detection of auditory stimuli in a patient with cerebral deafness. Cortex* 36(1), 71-80

2.5.4   External links

- *−751501308* at GPnotebook

2.6   Do not resuscitate

For the television episode, see Do Not Resuscitate (The Sopranos).

Do not resuscitate (DNR), or **no code**, is a legal order

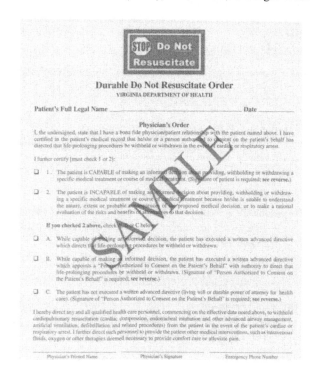

DNR form used in the Commonwealth of Virginia

written either in the hospital or on a legal form to withhold cardiopulmonary resuscitation (CPR) or advanced cardiac life support (ACLS), in respect of the wishes of a patient in case their heart were to stop or they were to stop breathing. "No code" is a reference to the use of "code" as jargon for "calling in a Code Blue" to alert a hospital's resuscitation team. The DNR request is usually made by the patient or health care power of attorney and allows the medical teams taking care of them to respect their wishes. In the health care community, allow natural death (AND), is a term that is quickly gaining favor as it focuses on what is being done, not what is being avoided. Some criticize the term "do not resuscitate" because it sounds as if something important is being withheld, while research shows that only about 5% of patients who require CPR outside the hospital and only 15% of patients who require CPR while in the hospital survive.[1][2] Patients who are elderly, are living in nursing homes, have multiple medical problems, or who have advanced cancer are much less likely to survive.[3]

A DNR does not affect any treatment other than that which would require intubation or CPR. Patients who are DNR can continue to get chemotherapy, antibiotics, dialysis, or any other appropriate treatments.

2.6.1 Alternative terms

Other terms and abbreviations for this order are used in different countries. *DNR* (Do Not Resuscitate) is a common abbreviation in the United States, Canada and the United Kingdom. It may be clarified in some regions with the addition of *DNI* (Do Not Intubate), although in some hospitals *DNR* alone will imply no intubation. Clinically, the vast majority of people requiring resuscitation will require intubation, making a DNI alone problematic.

Some areas of the United States and the United Kingdom include the letter A, as in *DNAR*, to clarify "Do Not *Attempt* Resuscitation." This alteration is so that it is not presumed by the patient or family that an attempt at resuscitation will be successful. Since the term DNR implies the omission of action, and therefore "giving up", some have advocated for these orders to be retermed *Allow Natural Death*.[4] New Zealand and Australia, and some hospitals in the UK, use the term *NFR* or *Not For Resuscitation*. Typically these abbreviations are not punctuated, e.g., *DNR* rather than *D.N.R.*

Another synonymous term is "*not to be resuscitated*" (*NTBR*).[5]

Until recently in the UK it was common to write "Not for 222" or conversationally, "Not for twos." This was implicitly a hospital DNR order, where 222 (or similar) is the hospital telephone number for the emergency resuscitation or crash team.

DNR compared with advance directive and living will

Advance directives and living wills are documents written by individuals themselves, so as to state their wishes for care, if they are no longer able to speak for themselves. In contrast, it is a physician or hospital staff member who writes a DNR "physician's order," based upon the wishes previously expressed by the individual in his or her advance directive or living will. Similarly, at a time when the individual is unable to express his wishes, but has previously used an advance directive to appoint an agent, then a physician can write such a DNR "physician's order" at the request of that individual's agent. These various situations are clearly enumerated in the "sample" DNR order presented on this page.

It should be stressed that, in the United States, an advance directive or living will is not sufficient to ensure a patient is treated under the DNR protocol, even if it is his wish, as neither an advance directive nor a living will is a legally binding document.

2.6.2 Usage by country

DNR documents are widespread in some countries and unavailable in others. In countries where a DNR is unavailable the decision to end resuscitation is made solely by physicians.

Middle East

DNRs are not recognized by Jordan. Physicians attempt to resuscitate all patients regardless of individual or familial wishes.[6] In Israel, it is possible to sign a DNR form as long as the patient is dying and aware of their actions.

United Kingdom

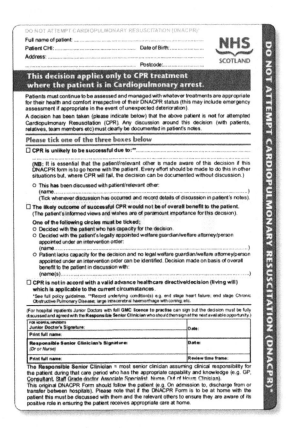

DNACPR form as used in Scotland

England and Wales In England and Wales, CPR is presumed in the event of a cardiac arrest unless a do not resuscitate order is in place. If they have capacity as defined under the Mental Capacity Act 2005 the patient may decline resuscitation, however any discussion is not in reference to consent to resuscitation and instead should be an explanation.[7] Patients may also specify their wishes and/or devolve their decision-making to a proxy using an advance directive, which are commonly referred to as 'Living Wills'. Patients and relatives cannot demand treatment (including CPR) which the doctor believes is futile and in this situation, it is their doctor's duty to act in their 'best interest', whether that means continuing or discontinuing treatment, using their clinical judgment. If they lack capacity relatives will often be asked for their opinion out of respect.

Scotland   In Scotland, the terminology used is "Do Not Attempt Cardiopulmonary Resuscitation" or "DNACPR". There is a single policy used across all of NHS Scotland. The legal standing is similar to that in England and Wales, in that CPR is viewed as a treatment and, although there is a general presumption that CPR will be performed in the case of cardiac arrest, this is not the case if it is viewed by the treating clinician to be futile. Patients and families cannot demand CPR to be performed if it is felt to be futile (as with any medical treatment) and a DNACPR can be issued despite disagreement, although it is good practice to involve all parties in the discussion.[8]

United States

In the United States the documentation is especially complicated in that each state accepts different forms, and advance directives and living wills are not accepted by EMS as legally valid forms. If a patient has a living will that states the patient wishes to be DNR but does not have an appropriately filled out state sponsored form that is co-signed by a physician, EMS will attempt resuscitation.

The DNR decision by patients was first litigated in 1976 in In re Quinlan. The New Jersey Supreme Court upheld the right of Karen Ann Quinlan's parents to order her removal from artificial ventilation. In 1991 Congress passed into law the Patient Self-Determination Act that mandated hospitals honor an individual's decision in their healthcare.[9] Forty-nine states currently permit the next of kin to make medical decisions of incapacitated relatives, the exception being Missouri. Missouri has a Living Will Statute that requires two witnesses to any signed advance directive that results in a DNR/DNI code status in the hospital.

In the U.S., cardiopulmonary resuscitation (CPR) and advanced cardiac life support (ACLS) will not be performed if a valid written "DNR" order is present. Many US states do not recognize living wills or health care proxies in the prehospital setting and prehospital personnel in those areas may be required to initiate resuscitation measures unless a specific state sponsored form is appropriately filled out and cosigned by a physician.[10][11]

Canada

Do not resuscitate orders are similar to those used in the United States. In 1995, the Canadian Medical Association, Canadian Hospital Association, Canadian Nursing Association, and Catholic Health Association of Canada worked with Canadian Bar Association clarify and create a **Joint Statement on Resuscitative Interventions** guideline for use to determine when and how DNR orders are assigned.[12] DNR orders must be discussed by doctors with the patient or patient agents or patient's significant others. Unilateral DNR by medical professionals can only be used if the patient is in a vegetative state.[12]

2.6.3   See also

- Advance Health Care Directive
- Cardiac arrest
- Power of attorney
- Letting die
- Euthanasia
- Uniform Rights of the Terminally Ill Act
- Patient Self-Determination Act
- Slow code

2.6.4   References

[1] PMID 17174021

[2] Zoch TW, Desbiens NA, DeStefano F, Stueland DT, Layde PM (July 2000). "Short- and long-term survival after cardiopulmonary resuscitation". *Arch. Intern. Med.* **160** (13): 1969–73. doi:10.1001/archinte.160.13.1969. PMID 10888971.

[3] Ehlenbach WJ, Barnato AE, Curtis JR, et al. (July 2009). "Epidemiologic study of in-hospital cardiopulmonary resuscitation in the elderly". *N. Engl. J. Med.* **361** (1): 22–31. doi:10.1056/NEJMoa0810245. PMC 2917337. PMID 19571280.

[4] Alternative to "DNR" Designation: "Allow Natural Death" - Making Sense in the Health Care Industry.

[5] Vincent JL, Van Vooren JP. [NTBR (Not to Be Resuscitated) in 10 questions]. Rev Med Brux. 2002 Dec;23(6):497-9. French. PubMed PMID 12584945.

[6] "Mideast med-school camp: divided by conflict, united by profession". *The Globe and Mail*. August 2009. Retrieved 2009-08-22. In hospitals in Jordan and Palestine, neither families nor social workers are allowed in the operating room

to observe resuscitation, says Mohamad Yousef, a sixth-year medical student from Jordan. There are also no DNRs. "If it was within the law, I would always work to save a patient, even if they didn't want me to," he says.

[7] "Decisions relating to cardiopulmonary resuscitation: A joint statement from the British Medical Association, the Resuscitation Council (UK) and the Royal College of Nursing" (PDF). *Resus.org.uk*. Resuscitation Council (UK). Retrieved 17 June 2014.

[8] Scottish Government (May 2010). "Do Not Attempt Cardiopulmonary Resuscitation (DNACPR): Integrated Adult Policy" (PDF). NHS Scotland.

[9] Eckberg, Evelyn (April 1998). "The continuing ethical dilemma of the do-not-resuscitate order". *AORN Journal*. Retrieved 2009-08-23. The right to refuse or terminate medical treatment began evolving in 1976 with the case of Karen Ann Quinlan v New Jersey (70NJ10, 355 A2d, 647 [NJ 1976]). This spawned subsequent cases leading to the use of the DNR order.(4) In 1991, the Patient Self-Determination Act mandated hospitals ensure that a patient's right to make personal health care decisions is upheld. According to the act, a patient has the right to refuse treatment, as well as the right to refuse resuscitative measures.(5) This right usually is accomplished by the use of the DNR order.

[10] "DO NOT RESUSCITATE – ADVANCE DIRECTIVES FOR EMS Frequently Asked Questions and Answers". *State of California Emergency Medical Services Authority*. 2007. Retrieved 2009-08-23. # What if the EMT cannot find the DNR form or evidence of a MedicAlert medallion? Will they withhold resuscitative measures if my family asks them to? No. EMS personnel are taught to proceed with CPR when needed, unless they are absolutely certain that a qualified DNR advance directive exists for that patient. If, after spending a reasonable (very short) amount of time looking for the form or medallion, they do not see it, they will proceed with lifesaving measures.

[11] "Frequently Asked Questions re: DNR's". *New York State Department of Health*. 1999-12-30. Retrieved 2009-08-23. May EMS providers accept living wills or health care proxies? A living will or health care proxy is NOT valid in the prehospital setting

[12] http://www.caringtotheend.ca/body.php?id=515&cc=1

2.6.5 External links

- Do Not Resuscitate Orders Published by the U.S. National Library of Medicine

- Decisions Relating to Cardiopulmonary Resuscitation Published by the Resuscitation Council (UK)

2.7 Electroencephalography

Not to be confused with other types of electrography.

Electroencephalography (**EEG**) is an electrophysiological monitoring method to record electrical activity of the brain. It is typically noninvasive, with the electrodes placed along the scalp, although invasive electrodes are sometimes used in specific applications. EEG measures voltage fluctuations resulting from ionic current within the neurons of the brain.[1] In clinical contexts, EEG refers to the recording of the brain's spontaneous electrical activity over a period of time,[1] as recorded from multiple electrodes placed on the scalp. Diagnostic applications generally focus on the spectral content of EEG, that is, the type of neural oscillations (popularly called "brain waves") that can be observed in EEG signals.

EEG is most often used to diagnose epilepsy, which causes abnormalities in EEG readings.[2] It is also used to diagnose sleep disorders, coma, encephalopathies, and brain death. EEG used to be a first-line method of diagnosis for tumors, stroke and other focal brain disorders,[3] but this use has decreased with the advent of high-resolution anatomical imaging techniques such as magnetic resonance imaging (MRI) and computed tomography (CT). Despite limited spatial resolution, EEG continues to be a valuable tool for research and diagnosis, especially when millisecond-range temporal resolution (not possible with CT or MRI) is required.

Derivatives of the EEG technique include evoked potentials (EP), which involves averaging the EEG activity time-locked to the presentation of a stimulus of some sort (visual, somatosensory, or auditory). Event-related potentials (ERPs) refer to averaged EEG responses that are time-locked to more complex processing of stimuli; this technique is used in cognitive science, cognitive psychology, and psychophysiological research.

2.7.1 Medical use

A routine clinical EEG recording typically lasts 20–30 minutes (plus preparation time) and usually involves recording from scalp electrodes. Routine EEG is typically used in the following clinical circumstances:

- to distinguish epileptic seizures from other types of spells, such as psychogenic non-epileptic seizures, syncope (fainting), sub-cortical movement disorders and migraine variants.

- to differentiate "organic" encephalopathy or delirium from primary psychiatric syndromes such as catatonia

- to serve as an adjunct test of brain death

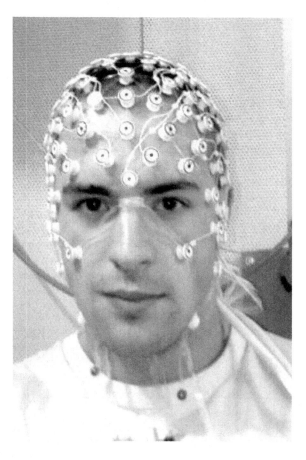

An EEG recording setup

- to characterize seizures for the purposes of treatment

- to localize the region of brain from which a seizure originates for work-up of possible seizure surgery

Additionally, EEG may be used to monitor certain procedures:

- to monitor the depth of anesthesia

- as an indirect indicator of cerebral perfusion in carotid endarterectomy

- to monitor amobarbital effect during the Wada test

EEG can also be used in intensive care units for brain function monitoring:

- to monitor for non-convulsive seizures/non-convulsive status epilepticus

- to monitor the effect of sedative/anesthesia in patients in medically induced coma (for treatment of refractory seizures or increased intracranial pressure)

- to monitor for secondary brain damage in conditions such as subarachnoid hemorrhage (currently a research method)

- to prognosticate, in certain instances, in patients with coma

- to determine whether to wean anti-epileptic medications

At times, a routine EEG is not sufficient, particularly when it is necessary to record a patient while he/she is having a seizure. In this case, the patient may be admitted to the hospital for days or even weeks, while EEG is constantly being recorded (along with time-synchronized video and audio recording). A recording of an actual seizure (i.e., an ictal recording, rather than an inter-ictal recording of a possibly epileptic patient at some period between seizures) can give significantly better information about whether or not a spell is an epileptic seizure and the focus in the brain from which the seizure activity emanates.

Epilepsy monitoring is typically done:

- to distinguish epileptic seizures from other types of spells, such as psychogenic non-epileptic seizures, syncope (fainting), sub-cortical movement disorders and migraine variants.

If a patient with epilepsy is being considered for resective surgery, it is often necessary to localize the focus (source) of the epileptic brain activity with a resolution greater than what is provided by scalp EEG. This is because the cerebrospinal fluid, skull and scalp *smear* the electrical potentials recorded by scalp EEG. In these cases, neurosurgeons typically implant strips and grids of electrodes (or penetrating depth electrodes) under the dura mater, through either a craniotomy or a burr hole. The recording of these signals is referred to as electrocorticography (ECoG), subdural EEG (sdEEG) or intracranial EEG (icEEG)--all terms for the same thing. The signal recorded from ECoG is on a different scale of activity than the brain activity recorded from scalp EEG. Low voltage, high frequency components that cannot be seen easily (or at all) in scalp EEG can be seen clearly in ECoG. Further, smaller electrodes (which cover a smaller parcel of brain surface) allow even lower voltage, faster components of brain activity to be seen. Some clinical sites record from penetrating microelectrodes.[1] EEG may be done in all pediatric patients presenting with first onset afebrile or complex febrile seizures.[4] EEG is not indicated for diagnosing headache.[5] Recurring headache is a common pain problem, and this procedure is sometimes used in a search for a diagnosis, but it has no advantage over routine clinical evaluation.[5]

2.7.2 Research use

EEG, and the related study of ERPs are used extensively in neuroscience, cognitive science, cognitive psychology, neurolinguistics and psychophysiological research. Many EEG techniques used in research are not standardized sufficiently for clinical use.

Advantages

Several other methods to study brain function exist, including functional magnetic resonance imaging (fMRI), positron emission tomography, magnetoencephalography (MEG), Nuclear magnetic resonance spectroscopy, Electrocorticography, Single-photon emission computed tomography, Near-infrared spectroscopy (NIRS), and Event-related optical signal (EROS). Despite the relatively poor spatial sensitivity of EEG, it possesses multiple advantages over some of these techniques:

- Hardware costs are significantly lower than those of most other techniques [6]

- EEG prevents limited availability of technologists to provide immediate care in high traffic hospitals.[7]

- EEG sensors can be used in more places than fMRI, SPECT, PET, MRS, or MEG, as these techniques require bulky and immobile equipment. For example, MEG requires equipment consisting of liquid helium-cooled detectors that can be used only in magnetically shielded rooms, altogether costing upwards of several million dollars;[8] and fMRI requires the use of a 1-ton magnet in, again, a shielded room.

- EEG has very high temporal resolution, on the order of milliseconds rather than seconds. EEG is commonly recorded at sampling rates between 250 and 2000 Hz in clinical and research settings, but modern EEG data collection systems are capable of recording at sampling rates above 20,000 Hz if desired. MEG and EROS are the only other noninvasive cognitive neuroscience techniques that acquire data at this level of temporal resolution.[8]

- EEG is relatively tolerant of subject movement, unlike most other neuroimaging techniques. There even exist methods for minimizing, and even eliminating movement artifacts in EEG data [9]

- EEG is silent, which allows for better study of the responses to auditory stimuli.

- EEG does not aggravate claustrophobia, unlike fMRI, PET, MRS, SPECT, and sometimes MEG[10]

- EEG does not involve exposure to high-intensity (>1 Tesla) magnetic fields, as in some of the other techniques, especially MRI and MRS. These can cause a variety of undesirable issues with the data, and also prohibit use of these techniques with participants that have metal implants in their body, such as metal-containing pacemakers[11]

- EEG does not involve exposure to radioligands, unlike positron emission tomography.[12]

- ERP studies can be conducted with relatively simple paradigms, compared with IE block-design fMRI studies

- Extremely uninvasive, unlike Electrocorticography, which actually requires electrodes to be placed on the surface of the brain.

EEG also has some characteristics that compare favorably with behavioral testing:

- EEG can detect covert processing (i.e., processing that does not require a response)[13]

- EEG can be used in subjects who are incapable of making a motor response[14]

- Some ERP components can be detected even when the subject is not attending to the stimuli

- Unlike other means of studying reaction time, ERPs can elucidate stages of processing (rather than just the final end result)[15]

- EEG is a powerful tool for tracking brain changes during different phases of life. EEG sleep analysis can indicate significant aspects of the timing of brain development, including evaluating adolescent brain maturation.[16] Brain activity can also be monitored by ct's.[17]

- In EEG there is a better understanding of what signal is measured as compared to other research techniques, i.e. the BOLD response in MRI.

Disadvantages

- Low spatial resolution on the scalp. fMRI, for example, can directly display areas of the brain that are active, while EEG requires intense interpretation just to hypothesize what areas are activated by a particular response.[18]

- EEG poorly measures neural activity that occurs below the upper layers of the brain (the cortex).

- Unlike PET and MRS, cannot identify specific locations in the brain at which various neurotransmitters, drugs, etc. can be found.[12]

- Often takes a long time to connect a subject to EEG, as it requires precise placement of dozens of electrodes around the head and the use of various gels, saline solutions, and/or pastes to keep them in place. While the length of time differs dependent on the specific EEG device used, as a general rule it takes considerably less time to prepare a subject for MEG, fMRI, MRS, and SPECT.

- Signal-to-noise ratio is poor, so sophisticated data analysis and relatively large numbers of subjects are needed to extract useful information from EEG[19]

With other neuroimaging techniques

Simultaneous EEG recordings and fMRI scans have been obtained successfully,[20][21] though successful simultaneous recording requires that several technical difficulties be overcome, such as the presence of ballistocardiographic artifact, MRI pulse artifact and the induction of electrical currents in EEG wires that move within the strong magnetic fields of the MRI. While challenging, these have been successfully overcome in a number of studies.[22]

MRI's produce detailed images created by generating strong magnetic fields that may induce potentially harmful displacement force and torque. These fields produce potentially harmful radio frequency heating and create image artifacts rendering images useless. Due to these potential risks, only certain medical devices can be used in an MR environment.

Similarly, simultaneous recordings with MEG and EEG have also been conducted, which has several advantages over using either technique alone:

- EEG requires accurate information about certain aspects of the skull that can only be estimated, such as skull radius, and conductivities of various skull locations. MEG does not have this issue, and a simultaneous analysis allows this to be corrected for.

- MEG and EEG both detect activity below the surface of the cortex very poorly, and like EEG, the level of error increases with the depth below the surface of the cortex one attempts to examine. However, the errors are very different between the techniques, and combining them thus allows for correction of some of this noise.

- MEG has access to virtually no sources of brain activity below a few centimetres under the cortex. EEG, on the other hand, can receive signals from greater depth, albeit with a high degree of noise. Combining the two makes it easier to determine what in the EEG signal comes from the surface (since MEG is very accurate in examining signals from the surface of the brain), and what comes from deeper in the brain, thus allowing for analysis of deeper brain signals than either EEG or MEG on its own.[23]

EEG has also been combined with positron emission tomography. This provides the advantage of allowing researchers to see what EEG signals are associated with different drug actions in the brain.[24]

2.7.3   Mechanisms

The brain's electrical charge is maintained by billions of neurons.[25] Neurons are electrically charged (or "polarized") by membrane transport proteins that pump ions across their membranes. Neurons are constantly exchanging ions with the extracellular milieu, for example to maintain resting potential and to propagate action potentials. Ions of similar charge repel each other, and when many ions are pushed out of many neurons at the same time, they can push their neighbours, who push their neighbours, and so on, in a wave. This process is known as volume conduction. When the wave of ions reaches the electrodes on the scalp, they can push or pull electrons on the metal on the electrodes. Since metal conducts the push and pull of electrons easily, the difference in push or pull voltages between any two electrodes can be measured by a voltmeter. Recording these voltages over time gives us the EEG.[26]

The electric potential generated by an individual neuron is far too small to be picked up by EEG or MEG.[27] EEG activity therefore always reflects the summation of the synchronous activity of thousands or millions of neurons that have similar spatial orientation. If the cells do not have similar spatial orientation, their ions do not line up and create waves to be detected. Pyramidal neurons of the cortex are thought to produce the most EEG signal because they are well-aligned and fire together. Because voltage fields fall off with the square of distance, activity from deep sources is more difficult to detect than currents near the skull.[28]

Scalp EEG activity shows oscillations at a variety of frequencies. Several of these oscillations have characteristic frequency ranges, spatial distributions and are associated with different states of brain functioning (e.g., waking and the various sleep stages). These oscillations represent synchronized activity over a network of neurons. The neuronal networks underlying some of these oscillations are understood (e.g., the thalamocortical resonance underlying sleep spindles), while many others are not (e.g., the system that generates the posterior basic rhythm). Research that measures both EEG and neuron spiking finds the relationship between the two is complex, with a combination of EEG power in the gamma band and phase in the delta band relating most strongly to neuron spike activity.[29]

2.7.4 Method

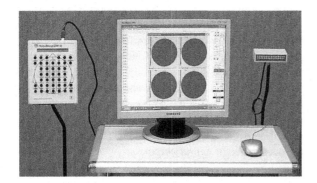

Computer Electroencephalograph Neurovisor-BMM 40

In conventional scalp EEG, the recording is obtained by placing electrodes on the scalp with a conductive gel or paste, usually after preparing the scalp area by light abrasion to reduce impedance due to dead skin cells. Many systems typically use electrodes, each of which is attached to an individual wire. Some systems use caps or nets into which electrodes are embedded; this is particularly common when high-density arrays of electrodes are needed.

Electrode locations and names are specified by the International 10–20 system[30] for most clinical and research applications (except when high-density arrays are used). This system ensures that the naming of electrodes is consistent across laboratories. In most clinical applications, 19 recording electrodes (plus ground and system reference) are used.[31] A smaller number of electrodes are typically used when recording EEG from neonates. Additional electrodes can be added to the standard set-up when a clinical or research application demands increased spatial resolution for a particular area of the brain. High-density arrays (typically via cap or net) can contain up to 256 electrodes more-or-less evenly spaced around the scalp.

Each electrode is connected to one input of a differential amplifier (one amplifier per pair of electrodes); a common system reference electrode is connected to the other input of each differential amplifier. These amplifiers amplify the voltage between the active electrode and the reference (typically 1,000–100,000 times, or 60–100 dB of voltage gain). In analog EEG, the signal is then filtered (next paragraph), and the EEG signal is output as the deflection of pens as paper passes underneath. Most EEG systems these days, however, are digital, and the amplified signal is digitized via an

analog-to-digital converter, after being passed through an anti-aliasing filter. Analog-to-digital sampling typically occurs at 256–512 Hz in clinical scalp EEG; sampling rates of up to 20 kHz are used in some research applications.

During the recording, a series of activation procedures may be used. These procedures may induce normal or abnormal EEG activity that might not otherwise be seen. These procedures include hyperventilation, photic stimulation (with a strobe light), eye closure, mental activity, sleep and sleep deprivation. During (inpatient) epilepsy monitoring, a patient's typical seizure medications may be withdrawn.

The digital EEG signal is stored electronically and can be filtered for display. Typical settings for the high-pass filter and a low-pass filter are 0.5-1 Hz and 35–70 Hz, respectively. The high-pass filter typically filters out slow artifact, such as electrogalvanic signals and movement artifact, whereas the low-pass filter filters out high-frequency artifacts, such as electromyographic signals. An additional notch filter is typically used to remove artifact caused by electrical power lines (60 Hz in the United States and 50 Hz in many other countries).[1]

The EEG signal can be processed by freely available EEG software such as EEGLAB or the Neurophysiological Biomarker Toolbox.

As part of an evaluation for epilepsy surgery, it may be necessary to insert electrodes near the surface of the brain, under the surface of the dura mater. This is accomplished via burr hole or craniotomy. This is referred to variously as "electrocorticography (ECoG)", "intracranial EEG (I-EEG)" or "subdural EEG (SD-EEG)". Depth electrodes may also be placed into brain structures, such as the amygdala or hippocampus, structures, which are common epileptic foci and may not be "seen" clearly by scalp EEG. The electrocorticographic signal is processed in the same manner as digital scalp EEG (above), with a couple of caveats. ECoG is typically recorded at higher sampling rates than scalp EEG because of the requirements of Nyquist theorem—the subdural signal is composed of a higher predominance of higher frequency components. Also, many of the artifacts that affect scalp EEG do not impact ECoG, and therefore display filtering is often not needed.

A typical adult human EEG signal is about 10 µV to 100 µV in amplitude when measured from the scalp[32] and is about 10–20 mV when measured from subdural electrodes.

Since an EEG voltage signal represents a difference between the voltages at two electrodes, the display of the EEG for the reading encephalographer may be set up in one of several ways. The representation of the EEG channels is referred to as a *montage*.

Sequential montage Each channel (i.e., waveform) represents the difference between two adjacent electrodes. The entire montage consists of a series of these channels. For example, the channel "Fp1-F3" represents the difference in voltage between the Fp1 electrode and the F3 electrode. The next channel in the montage, "F3-C3," represents the voltage difference between F3 and C3, and so on through the entire array of electrodes.

Referential montage Each channel represents the difference between a certain electrode and a designated reference electrode. There is no standard position for this reference; it is, however, at a different position than the "recording" electrodes. Midline positions are often used because they do not amplify the signal in one hemisphere vs. the other. Another popular reference is "linked ears," which is a physical or mathematical average of electrodes attached to both earlobes or mastoids.

Average reference montage The outputs of all of the amplifiers are summed and averaged, and this averaged signal is used as the common reference for each channel.

Laplacian montage Each channel represents the difference between an electrode and a weighted average of the surrounding electrodes.[33]

When analog (paper) EEGs are used, the technologist switches between montages during the recording in order to highlight or better characterize certain features of the EEG. With digital EEG, all signals are typically digitized and stored in a particular (usually referential) montage; since any montage can be constructed mathematically from any other, the EEG can be viewed by the electroencephalographer in any display montage that is desired.

The EEG is read by a clinical neurophysiologist or neurologist (depending on local custom and law regarding medical specialities), optimally one who has specific training in the interpretation of EEGs for clinical purposes. This is done by visual inspection of the waveforms, called graphoelements. The use of computer signal processing of the EEG—so-called Quantitative electroencephalography—is somewhat controversial when used for clinical purposes (although there are many research uses).

Limitations

EEG has several limitations. Most important is its poor spatial resolution.[34] EEG is most sensitive to a particular set of post-synaptic potentials: those generated in superficial layers of the cortex, on the crests of gyri directly abutting the skull and radial to the skull. Dendrites, which are deeper in the cortex, inside sulci, in midline or deep structures (such as the cingulate gyrus or hippocampus), or producing currents that are tangential to the skull, have far less contribution to the EEG signal.

EEG recordings do not directly capture axonal action potentials. An action potential can be accurately represented as a current quadrupole, meaning that the resulting field decreases more rapidly than the ones produced by the current dipole of post-synaptic potentials.[35] In addition, since EEGs represent averages of thousands of neurons, a large population of cells in synchronous activity is necessary to cause a significant deflection on the recordings. Action potentials are very fast and, as a consequence, the chances of field summation are slim. However, neural backpropagation, as a typically longer dendritic current dipole, can be picked up by EEG electrodes and is a reliable indication of the occurrence of neural output.

Not only do EEGs capture dendritic currents almost exclusively as opposed to axonal currents, they also show a preference for activity on populations of parallel dendrites and transmitting current in the same direction at the same time. Pyramidal neurons of cortical layers II/III and V extend apical dendrites to layer I. Currents moving up or down these processes underlie most of the signals produced by electroencephalography.[36]

Therefore, EEG provides information with a large bias to select neuron types, and generally should not be used to make claims about global brain activity. The meninges, cerebrospinal fluid and skull "smear" the EEG signal, obscuring its intracranial source.

It is mathematically impossible to reconstruct a unique intracranial current source for a given EEG signal,[1] as some currents produce potentials that cancel each other out. This is referred to as the inverse problem. However, much work has been done to produce remarkably good estimates of, at least, a localized electric dipole that represents the recorded currents.

EEG vs fMRI, fNIRS and PET

EEG has several strong points as a tool for exploring brain activity. EEGs can detect changes over milliseconds, which is excellent considering an action potential takes approximately 0.5-130 milliseconds to propagate across a single neuron, depending on the type of neuron.[37] Other methods of looking at brain activity, such as PET and fMRI have time resolution between seconds and minutes. EEG measures the brain's electrical activity directly, while other methods record changes in blood flow (e.g., SPECT, fMRI) or metabolic activity (e.g., PET, NIRS), which are indirect markers of brain electrical activity. EEG can be used simultaneously with fMRI so that high-temporal-resolution data can be recorded at the same time as high-spatial-resolution data, however, since the data derived from each occurs over a different time course, the data sets do not necessarily represent exactly the same brain activity. There are technical difficulties associated with combining these two modalities, including the need to remove the *MRI gradient artifact* present during MRI acquisition and the ballistocardiographic artifact (resulting from the pulsatile motion of blood and tissue) from the EEG. Furthermore, currents can be induced in moving EEG electrode wires due to the magnetic field of the MRI.

EEG can be used simultaneously with NIRS without major technical difficulties. There is no influence of these modalities on each other and a combined measurement can give useful information about electrical activity as well as local hemodynamics.

EEG vs MEG

EEG reflects correlated synaptic activity caused by post-synaptic potentials of cortical neurons. The ionic currents involved in the generation of fast action potentials may not contribute greatly to the averaged field potentials representing the EEG .[27][38] More specifically, the scalp electrical potentials that produce EEG are generally thought to be caused by the extracellular ionic currents caused by dendritic electrical activity, whereas the fields producing magnetoencephalographic signals[8] are associated with intracellular ionic currents .[39]

EEG can be recorded at the same time as MEG so that data from these complementary high-time-resolution techniques can be combined.

Studies on numerical modeling of EEG and MEG have also been done.[40]

2.7.5 Normal activity

- One second of EEG signal

- The sample of human EEG with prominent resting state activity - alpha-rhythm. Left - EEG traces (horizontal - time in seconds; vertical - amplitudes, scale 100uV). Right - power spectra of shown signals (vertical lines - 10 and 20Hz, scale is linear). Alpha-rhythm consists of sinusoidal-like waves with frequencies in 8-12Hz range (11Hz in this case) more prominent in posterior sites. Alpha range is red at power spectrum graph.

- The sample of human EEG with in resting state. Left - EEG traces (horizontal - time in seconds; vertical

- amplitudes, scale 100uV). Right - power spectra of shown signals (vertical lines - 10 and 20Hz, scale is linear). 80-90% of people have prominent sinusoidal-like waves with frequencies in 8-12Hz range - alpha rhythm. Others (like this) lack this type of activity.

- The samples of main types of artifacts in human EEG. 1 - Electrooculographic artifact caused by the excitation of eyeball's muscles (related to blinking, for example). Big amplitude, slow, positive wave prominent in frontal electrodes. 2 - Electrode's artifact caused by bad contact (and thus bigger impedance) between P3 electrode and skin. 3 - Swallowing artifact. 4 - Common reference electrode's artifact caused by bad contact between reference electrode and skin. Huge wave similar in all channels.

The EEG is typically described in terms of (1) rhythmic activity and (2) transients. The rhythmic activity is divided into bands by frequency. To some degree, these frequency bands are a matter of nomenclature (i.e., any rhythmic activity between 8–12 Hz can be described as "alpha"), but these designations arose because rhythmic activity within a certain frequency range was noted to have a certain distribution over the scalp or a certain biological significance. Frequency bands are usually extracted using spectral methods (for instance Welch) as implemented for instance in freely available EEG software such as EEGLAB or the Neurophysiological Biomarker Toolbox. Computational processing of the EEG is often named Quantitative electroencephalography (qEEG).

Most of the cerebral signal observed in the scalp EEG falls in the range of 1–20 Hz (activity below or above this range is likely to be artifactual, under standard clinical recording techniques). Waveforms are subdivided into bandwidths known as alpha, beta, theta, and delta to signify the majority of the EEG used in clinical practice.[41]

The practice of using only whole numbers in the definitions comes from practical considerations in the days when only whole cycles could be counted on paper records. This leads to gaps in the definitions, as seen elsewhere on this page. The theoretical definitions have always been more carefully defined to include all frequencies. Unfortunately there is no agreement in standard reference works on what these ranges should be - values for the upper end of alpha and lower end of beta include 12,13,14 and 15.If the threshold is taken as 14 Hz, then the slowest beta wave has about the same duration as the longest spike (70ms) which makes this the most useful value.

Others sometimes divide the bands into sub bands for the purposes of data analysis.

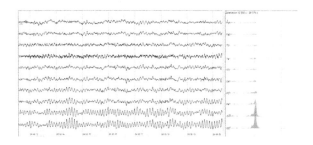

Human EEG with prominent alpha-rhythm

Wave patterns

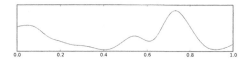

delta waves.

- Delta is the frequency range up to 4 Hz. It tends to be the highest in amplitude and the slowest waves. It is seen normally in adults in slow wave sleep. It is also seen normally in babies. It may occur focally with subcortical lesions and in general distribution with diffuse lesions, metabolic encephalopathy hydrocephalus or deep midline lesions. It is usually most prominent frontally in adults (e.g. FIRDA - Frontal Intermittent Rhythmic Delta) and posteriorly in children (e.g. OIRDA - Occipital Intermittent Rhythmic Delta).

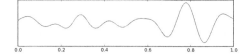

theta waves.

- Theta is the frequency range from 4 Hz to 7 Hz. Theta is seen normally in young children. It may be seen in drowsiness or arousal in older children and adults; it can also be seen in meditation.[48] Excess theta for age represents abnormal activity. It can be seen as a focal disturbance in focal subcortical lesions; it can be seen in generalized distribution in diffuse disorder or metabolic encephalopathy or deep midline disorders or some instances of hydrocephalus. On the contrary this range has been associated with reports of relaxed, meditative, and creative states.

- Alpha is the frequency range from 7 Hz to 14 Hz. Hans Berger named the first rhythmic EEG activity he saw

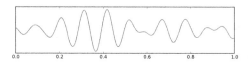

alpha waves.

as the "alpha wave". This was the "posterior basic rhythm" (also called the "posterior dominant rhythm" or the "posterior alpha rhythm"), seen in the posterior regions of the head on both sides, higher in amplitude on the dominant side. It emerges with closing of the eyes and with relaxation, and attenuates with eye opening or mental exertion. The posterior basic rhythm is actually slower than 8 Hz in young children (therefore technically in the theta range). In addition

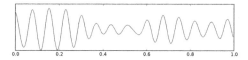

sensorimotor rhythm aka mu rhythm.

to the posterior basic rhythm, there are other normal alpha rhythms such as the mu rhythm (alpha activity in the contralateral sensory and motor cortical areas) that emerges when the hands and arms are idle; and the "third rhythm" (alpha activity in the temporal or frontal lobes).[49][50] Alpha can be abnormal; for example, an EEG that has diffuse alpha occurring in coma and is not responsive to external stimuli is referred to as "alpha coma".

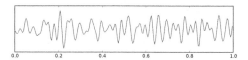

beta waves.

- Beta is the frequency range from 15 Hz to about 30 Hz. It is seen usually on both sides in symmetrical distribution and is most evident frontally. Beta activity is closely linked to motor behavior and is generally attenuated during active movements.[51] Low amplitude beta with multiple and varying frequencies is often associated with active, busy or anxious thinking and active concentration. Rhythmic beta with a dominant set of frequencies is associated with various pathologies and drug effects, especially benzodiazepines. It may be absent or reduced in areas of cortical damage. It is the dominant rhythm in patients who are alert or anxious or who have their eyes open.

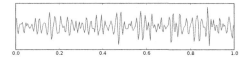

gamma waves.

- Gamma is the frequency range approximately 30–100 Hz. Gamma rhythms are thought to represent binding of different populations of neurons together into a network for the purpose of carrying out a certain cognitive or motor function.[1]

- Mu ranges 8–13 Hz., and partly overlaps with other frequencies. It reflects the synchronous firing of motor neurons in rest state. Mu suppression is thought to reflect motor mirror neuron systems, because when an action is observed, the pattern extinguishes, possibly because of the normal neuronal system and the mirror neuron system "go out of sync", and interfere with each other.[46]

"Ultra-slow" or "near-DC" (Direct current) activity is recorded using DC amplifiers in some research contexts. It is not typically recorded in a clinical context because the signal at these frequencies is susceptible to a number of artifacts.

Some features of the EEG are transient rather than rhythmic. Spikes and sharp waves may represent seizure activity or interictal activity in individuals with epilepsy or a predisposition toward epilepsy. Other transient features are normal: vertex waves and sleep spindles are seen in normal sleep.

Note that there are types of activity that are statistically uncommon, but not associated with dysfunction or disease. These are often referred to as "normal variants." The mu rhythm is an example of a normal variant.

The normal Electroencephalography (EEG) varies by age. The neonatal EEG is quite different from the adult EEG. The EEG in childhood generally has slower frequency oscillations than the adult EEG.

The normal EEG also varies depending on state. The EEG is used along with other measurements (EOG, EMG) to define sleep stages in polysomnography. Stage I sleep (equivalent to drowsiness in some systems) appears on the EEG as drop-out of the posterior basic rhythm. There can be an increase in theta frequencies. Santamaria and Chiappa cataloged a number of the variety of patterns associated with drowsiness. Stage II sleep is characterized by sleep spindles—transient runs of rhythmic activity in the 12–14 Hz range (sometimes referred to as the "sigma" band) that have a frontal-central maximum. Most of the activity in

Stage II is in the 3–6 Hz range. Stage III and IV sleep are defined by the presence of delta frequencies and are often referred to collectively as "slow-wave sleep." Stages I-IV comprise non-REM (or "NREM") sleep. The EEG in REM (rapid eye movement) sleep appears somewhat similar to the awake EEG.

EEG under general anesthesia depends on the type of anesthetic employed. With halogenated anesthetics, such as halothane or intravenous agents, such as propofol, a rapid (alpha or low beta), nonreactive EEG pattern is seen over most of the scalp, especially anteriorly; in some older terminology this was known as a WAR (widespread anterior rapid) pattern, contrasted with a WAIS (widespread slow) pattern associated with high doses of opiates. Anesthetic effects on EEG signals are beginning to be understood at the level of drug actions on different kinds of synapses and the circuits that allow synchronized neuronal activity (see: http://www.stanford.edu/group/maciverlab/).

2.7.6 Artifacts

Biological artifacts

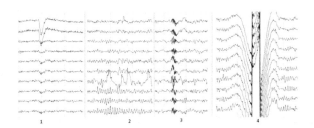

Main types of artifacts in human EEG

Electrical signals detected along the scalp by an EEG, but that originate from non-cerebral origin are called artifacts. EEG data is almost always contaminated by such artifacts. The amplitude of artifacts can be quite large relative to the size of amplitude of the cortical signals of interest. This is one of the reasons why it takes considerable experience to correctly interpret EEGs clinically. Some of the most common types of biological artifacts include:

- Eye-induced artifacts (includes eye blinks, eye movements and extra-ocular muscle activity)

- ECG (cardiac) artifacts

- EMG (muscle activation)-induced artifacts

- Glossokinetic artifacts

The most prominent eye-induced artifacts are caused by the potential difference between the cornea and retina, which is quite large compared to cerebral potentials. When the eyes and eyelids are completely still, this corneo-retinal dipole does not affect EEG. However, blinks occur several times per minute, the eyes movements occur several times per second. Eyelid movements, occurring mostly during blinking or vertical eye movements, elicit a large potential seen mostly in the difference between the Electrooculography (EOG) channels above and below the eyes. An established explanation of this potential regards the eyelids as sliding electrodes that short-circuit the positively charged cornea to the extra-ocular skin.[52][53] Rotation of the eyeballs, and consequently of the corneo-retinal dipole, increases the potential in electrodes towards which the eyes are rotated, and decrease the potentials in the opposing electrodes.[54] Eye movements called saccades also generate transient electromyographic potentials, known as saccadic spike potentials (SPs).[55] The spectrum of these SPs overlaps the gamma-band (see Gamma wave), and seriously confounds analysis of induced gamma-band responses,[56] requiring tailored artifact correction approaches.[55] Purposeful or reflexive eye blinking also generates electromyographic potentials, but more importantly there is reflexive movement of the eyeball during blinking that gives a characteristic artifactual appearance of the EEG (see Bell's phenomenon).

Eyelid fluttering artifacts of a characteristic type were previously called Kappa rhythm (or Kappa waves). It is usually seen in the prefrontal leads, that is, just over the eyes. Sometimes they are seen with mental activity. They are usually in the Theta (4–7 Hz) or Alpha (7–14 Hz) range. They were named because they were believed to originate from the brain. Later study revealed they were generated by rapid fluttering of the eyelids, sometimes so minute that it was difficult to see. They are in fact noise in the EEG reading, and should not technically be called a rhythm or wave. Therefore, current usage in electroencephalography refers to the phenomenon as an eyelid fluttering artifact, rather than a Kappa rhythm (or wave).[57]

Some of these artifacts can be useful in various applications. The EOG signals, for instance, can be used to detect[55] and track eye-movements, which are very important in polysomnography, and is also in conventional EEG for assessing possible changes in alertness, drowsiness or sleep.

ECG artifacts are quite common and can be mistaken for spike activity. Because of this, modern EEG acquisition commonly includes a one-channel ECG from the extremities. This also allows the EEG to identify cardiac arrhythmias that are an important differential diagnosis to syncope or other episodic/attack disorders.

Glossokinetic artifacts are caused by the potential difference between the base and the tip of the tongue. Minor tongue movements can contaminate the EEG, especially in parkinsonian and tremor disorders.

Environmental artifacts

In addition to artifacts generated by the body, many artifacts originate from outside the body. Movement by the patient, or even just settling of the electrodes, may cause *electrode pops*, spikes originating from a momentary change in the impedance of a given electrode. Poor grounding of the EEG electrodes can cause significant 50 or 60 Hz artifact, depending on the local power system's frequency. A third source of possible interference can be the presence of an IV drip; such devices can cause rhythmic, fast, low-voltage bursts, which may be confused for spikes.

Artifact correction

Recently, independent component analysis (ICA) techniques have been used to correct or remove EEG contaminants.[55][58][59][60][61][62] These techniques attempt to "unmix" the EEG signals into some number of underlying components. There are many source separation algorithms, often assuming various behaviors or natures of EEG. Regardless, the principle behind any particular method usually allow "remixing" only those components that would result in "clean" EEG by nullifying (zeroing) the weight of unwanted components. Fully automated artifact rejection methods, which use ICA, have also been developed.[63]

In the last few years, by comparing data from paralysed and unparalysed subjects, EEG contamination by muscle has been shown to be far more prevalent than had previously been realized, particularly in the gamma range above 20 Hz.[64] However, Surface Laplacian has been shown to be effective in eliminating muscle artefact, particularly for central electrodes, which are further from the strongest contaminants.[65] The combination of Surface Laplacian with automated techniques for removing muscle components using ICA proved particularly effective in a follow up study.[66]

2.7.7   Abnormal activity

Abnormal activity can broadly be separated into epileptiform and non-epileptiform activity. It can also be separated into focal or diffuse.

Focal epileptiform discharges represent fast, synchronous potentials in a large number of neurons in a somewhat discrete area of the brain. These can occur as interictal activity, between seizures, and represent an area of cortical irritability that may be predisposed to producing epileptic seizures. Interictal discharges are not wholly reliable for determining whether a patient has epilepsy nor where his/her seizure might originate. (See focal epilepsy.)

Generalized epileptiform discharges often have an anterior maximum, but these are seen synchronously throughout the entire brain. They are strongly suggestive of a generalized epilepsy.

Focal non-epileptiform abnormal activity may occur over areas of the brain where there is focal damage of the cortex or white matter. It often consists of an increase in slow frequency rhythms and/or a loss of normal higher frequency rhythms. It may also appear as focal or unilateral decrease in amplitude of the EEG signal.

Diffuse non-epileptiform abnormal activity may manifest as diffuse abnormally slow rhythms or bilateral slowing of normal rhythms, such as the PBR.

Intracortical Encephalogram electrodes and sub-dural electrodes can be used in tandem to discriminate and discretize artifact from epileptiform and other severe neurological events.

More advanced measures of abnormal EEG signals have also recently received attention as possible biomarkers for different disorders such as Alzheimer's disease.[67]

Remote communication

The United States Army Research Office budgeted $4 million in 2009 to researchers at the University of California, Irvine to develop EEG processing techniques to identify correlates of imagined speech and intended direction to enable soldiers on the battlefield to communicate via computer-mediated reconstruction of team members' EEG signals, in the form of understandable signals such as words.[68]

2.7.8 Economics

Inexpensive EEG devices exist for the low-cost research and consumer markets. Recently, a few companies have miniaturized medical grade EEG technology to create versions accessible to the wider public. Some of these companies have even built commercial EEG devices retailing for less than $100 USD.

- In 2004 OpenEEG released its ModularEEG as open source hardware. Compatible open source software includes a game for balancing a ball.

- In 2007 NeuroSky released the first affordable consumer based EEG along with the game NeuroBoy. This was also the first large scale EEG device to use dry sensor technology.[69]

- In 2008 OCZ Technology developed device for use in video games relying primarily on electromyography.

- In 2008 the Final Fantasy developer Square Enix announced that it was partnering with NeuroSky to create a game, Judecca.[70][71]

- In 2009 Mattel partnered with NeuroSky to release the Mindflex, a game that used an EEG to steer a ball through an obstacle course. By far the best selling consumer based EEG to date.[70][72]

- In 2009 Uncle Milton Industries partnered with NeuroSky to release the Star Wars Force Trainer, a game designed to create the illusion of possessing The Force.[70][73]

- In 2009 Emotiv released the EPOC, a 14 channel EEG device. The EPOC is the first commercial BCI to not use dry sensor technology, requiring users to apply a saline solution to electrode pads (which need remoistening after an hour or two of use).[74]

- In 2010, NeuroSky added a blink and electromyography function to the MindSet.[75]

- In 2011, NeuroSky released the MindWave, an EEG device designed for educational purposes and games.[76] The MindWave won the Guinness Book of World Records award for "Heaviest machine moved using a brain control interface".[77]

- In 2011, Rhythmlink released Disposable Webbed™ EEG Electrodes, a flat, single-use EEG electrode. The Webbed Electrode provides a greater surface area to provide more area to be in contact with conductive material and a more comfortable experience for the patient.

- In 2012, a Japanese gadget project, neurowear, released Necomimi: a headset with motorized cat ears. The headset is a NeuroSky MindWave unit with two motors on the headband where a cat's ears might be. Slipcovers shaped like cat ears sit over the motors so that as the device registers emotional states the ears move to relate. For example, when relaxed, the ears fall to the sides and perk up again when excited.

- In 2014, OpenBCI released an eponymous Open Source brain-computer interface after a successful kickstarter campaign in 2013. The basic OpenBCI has 8 channels, expandable to 16, and supports EEG, EKG, and EMG. The OpenBCI is based on the Texas Instruments ADS1299 IC and the Arduino or PIC microcontroller, and costs $399 for the basic version. It uses standard metal cup electrodes and conductive paste.

- In 2014, HyperNeuro released a wearable EEG head-set. The basic headset has only 1 channel, due to high performance active electrode, it can measure mental state accurately.[Citation Needed]

- in 2015, mind solutions inc released the smallest consumer bci to date, the neurosync. A powerful single dry sensor eeg no bigger than a Bluetooth ear piece

[78]

2.7.9   History

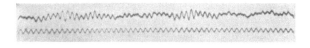

The first human EEG recording obtained by Hans Berger in 1924. The upper tracing is EEG, and the lower is a 10 Hz timing signal.

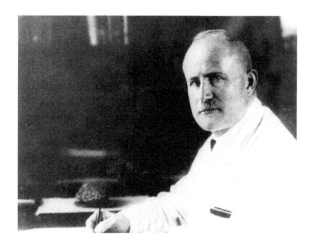

Hans Berger

The following history of EEG is detailed by Barbara E. Swartz in *Electroencephalography and Clinical Neurophysiology*.[79] In 1875, Richard Caton (1842–1926), a physician practicing in Liverpool, presented his findings about electrical phenomena of the exposed cerebral hemispheres of rabbits and monkeys in the *British Medical Journal*. In 1890, Polish physiologist Adolf Beck published an investigation of spontaneous electrical activity of the brain of rabbits and dogs that included rhythmic oscillations altered by light. Beck started experiments on the electrical brain activity of animals. Beck placed electrodes directly on the surface of brain to test for sensory stimulation. His observation of fluctuating brain activity lead to the conclusion of brain waves.[80]

In 1912, Ukrainian physiologist Vladimir Vladimirovich Pravdich-Neminsky published the first animal EEG and

the evoked potential of the mammalian (dog).[81] In 1914, Napoleon Cybulski and Jelenska-Macieszyna photographed EEG recordings of experimentally induced seizures.

German physiologist and psychiatrist Hans Berger (1873–1941) recorded the first human EEG in 1924.[82] Expanding on work previously conducted on animals by Richard Caton and others, Berger also invented the electroencephalogram (giving the device its name), an invention described "as one of the most surprising, remarkable, and momentous developments in the history of clinical neurology".[83] His discoveries were first confirmed by British scientists Edgar Douglas Adrian and B. H. C. Matthews in 1934 and developed by them.

In 1934, Fisher and Lowenback first demonstrated epileptiform spikes. In 1935 Gibbs, Davis and Lennox described interictal spike waves and the three cycles/s pattern of clinical absence seizures, which began the field of clinical electroencephalography. Subsequently, in 1936 Gibbs and Jasper reported the interictal spike as the focal signature of epilepsy. The same year, the first EEG laboratory opened at Massachusetts General Hospital.

Franklin Offner (1911–1999), professor of biophysics at Northwestern University developed a prototype of the EEG that incorporated a piezoelectric inkwriter called a Crystograph (the whole device was typically known as the Offner Dynograph).

In 1947, The American EEG Society was founded and the first International EEG congress was held. In 1953 Aserinsky and Kleitman described REM sleep.

In the 1950s, William Grey Walter developed an adjunct to EEG called EEG topography, which allowed for the mapping of electrical activity across the surface of the brain. This enjoyed a brief period of popularity in the 1980s and seemed especially promising for psychiatry. It was never accepted by neurologists and remains primarily a research tool.

2.7.10   Future research

The EEG has been used for many purposes besides the conventional uses of clinical diagnosis and conventional cognitive neuroscience. An early use was during World War II by the U.S. Army Air Corps to screen out pilots in danger of having seizures;[84] long-term EEG recordings in epilepsy patients are still used today for seizure prediction. Neurofeedback remains an important extension, and in its most advanced form is also attempted as the basis of brain computer interfaces. The EEG is also used quite extensively in the field of neuromarketing. In recent years, researchers have relied on EEG to understand the neural basis of swallowing.[85]

The EEG is altered by drugs that affect brain functions, the chemicals that are the basis for psychopharmacology. Berger's early experiments recorded the effects of drugs on EEG. The science of pharmaco-electroencephalography has developed methods to identify substances that systematically alter brain functions for therapeutic and recreational use.

Honda is attempting to develop a system to enable an operator to control its Asimo robot using EEG, a technology it eventually hopes to incorporate into its automobiles.[86]

EEGs have been used as an evidence in criminal trials in the Indian state of Maharastra.[87][88]

2.7.11 See also

- 10-20 system (EEG)

- Binaural beats

- Brain-computer interface

- Brainwave synchronization

- CAET-Canadian association of EEG Technology

- Comparison of consumer brain-computer interface devices

- Direct brain interfaces

- EEG measures during anesthesia

- EEG microstates

- Electrocorticography

- Electromagnetic Weapon

- Electroneurogram

- Electropalatograph

- Emotiv Systems

- European data format

- Event-related potential

- Evoked potential

- FieldTrip

- God helmet

- Hemoencephalography

- Hypersynchronization of electrophysiological activity in epilepsy

- Imagined Speech

- Induced activity

- Intracranial EEG

- Local field potentials

- Magnetoencephalography

- Mind machine

- Neural oscillations

- Neurofeedback

- Ongoing brain activity

- Spontaneous potential

2.7.12 References

[1] Niedermeyer E. and da Silva F.L. (2004). *Electroencephalography: Basic Principles, Clinical Applications, and Related Fields*. Lippincot Williams & Wilkins. ISBN 0-7817-5126-8.

[2] *Atlas of EEG & Seizure Semiology*. B. Abou-Khalil; Musilus, K.E.; Elsevier, 2006.

[3] "EEG".

[4] Dr Mohammed Ashfaque Tinmaswala, Dr Valinjker S.K, Dr Shilpa Hegde, Dr Parmeshwar Taware Electroencephalographic Abnormalities in First Onset Afebrile and Complex Febrile Seizures and Its Association with Type of Seizures. http://jmscr.igmpublication.org/v3-i8/28%20jmscr.pdf

[5] American Academy of Neurology. "Five Things Physicians and Patients Should Question". *Choosing Wisely: an initiative of the ABIM Foundation* (American Academy of Neurology). Retrieved August 1, 2013, which cites

- Gronseth, G. S.; Greenberg, M. K. (1995). "The utility of the electroencephalogram in the evaluation of patients presenting with headache: A review of the literature". *Neurology* **45** (7): 1263–1267. doi:10.1212/WNL.45.7.1263. PMID 7617180.

[6] Vespa, Paul M.; Nenov, Val; Nuwer, Marc R. (1999). "Continuous EEG Monitoring in the Intensive Care Unit: Early Findings and Clinical Efficacy". *Journal of Clinical Neurophysiology* **16** (1): 1–13. doi:10.1097/00004691-199901000-00001. PMID 10082088.

[7] Schultz, Teal L. (2012). "Technical Tips: MRI Compatible EEG Electrodes: Advantages, Disadvantages, And Financial Feasibility In A Clinical Setting.". *Neurodiagnostic Journal* *52.1*: 69–81.

[8] Hämäläinen, Matti; Hari, Riitta; Ilmoniemi, Risto J.; Knuutila, Jukka; Lounasmaa, Olli V. (1993). "Magnetoencephalography-theory, instrumentation, and applications to noninvasive studies of the working human brain". *Reviews of Modern Physics* **65** (2): 413–97. Bibcode:1993RvMP...65..413H. doi:10.1103/RevModPhys.65.413.

[9] O'Regan, S; Faul, S; Marnane, W (2010). "2010 Annual International Conference of the IEEE Engineering in Medicine and Biology". pp. 6353–6. doi:10.1109/IEMBS.2010.5627282. ISBN 978-1-4244-4123-5. |chapter= ignored (help)

[10] Murphy, Kieran J.; Brunberg, James A. (1997). "Adult claustrophobia, anxiety and sedation in MRI". *Magnetic Resonance Imaging* **15** (1): 51–4. doi:10.1016/S0730-725X(96)00351-7. PMID 9084025.

[11] Schenck, John F. (1996). "The role of magnetic susceptibility in magnetic resonance imaging: MRI magnetic compatibility of the first and second kinds". *Medical Physics* **23** (6): 815–50. doi:10.1118/1.597854. PMID 8798169.

[12] Yasuno, Fumihiko; Brown, Amira K; Zoghbi, Sami S; Krushinski, Joseph H; Chernet, Eyassu; Tauscher, Johannes; Schaus, John M; Phebus, Lee A; Chesterfield, Amy K; Felder, Christian C; Gladding, Robert L; Hong, Jinsoo; Halldin, Christer; Pike, Victor W; Innis, Robert B (2007). "The PET Radioligand \11C]MePPEP Binds Reversibly and with High Specific Signal to Cannabinoid CB1 Receptors in Nonhuman Primate Brain". *Neuropsychopharmacology* **33** (2): 259–69. doi:10.1038/sj.npp.1301402. PMID 17392732.

[13] Mulholland, Thomas (2012). "Objective EEG Methods for Studying Covert Shifts of Visual Attention". In McGuigan, F. J.; Schoonover, R. A. *The Psychophysiology of Thinking: Studies of Covert Processes*. pp. 109–51. ISBN 978-0-323-14700-2.

[14] Hinterberger, Thilo; Kübler, Andrea; Kaiser, Jochen; Neumann, Nicola; Birbaumer, Niels (2003). "A brain–computer interface (BCI) for the locked-in: Comparison of different EEG classifications for the thought translation device". *Clinical Neurophysiology* **114** (3): 416–25. doi:10.1016/S1388-2457(02)00411-X. PMID 12705422.

[15] Sereno, SC; Rayner, K; Posner, MI (1998). "Establishing a time-line of word recognition: Evidence from eye movements and event-related potentials". *NeuroReport* **9** (10): 2195–200. doi:10.1097/00001756-199807130-00009. PMID 9694199.

[16] Feinberg, I.; Campbell, I. G. (2012). "Longitudinal sleep EEG trajectories indicate complex patterns of adolescent brain maturation". *AJP: Regulatory, Integrative and Comparative Physiology* **304** (4): R296–303. doi:10.1152/ajpregu.00422.2012. PMC 3567357. PMID 23193115. Lay summary – *ScienceDaily* (March 19, 2013).

[17] http://www.ct.gov/ceq/cwp/view.asp?a=987&q=249438[]

[18] Srinivasan, Ramesh (1999). "Methods to Improve the Spatial Resolution of EEG". *International Journal* **1** (1): 102–11.

[19] Schlögl, Alois; Slater, Mel; Pfurtscheller, Gert (2002). "Presence research and EEG" (PDF).

[20] Horovitz, Silvina G.; Skudlarski, Pawel; Gore, John C. (2002). "Correlations and dissociations between BOLD signal and P300 amplitude in an auditory oddball task: A parametric approach to combining fMRI and ERP". *Magnetic Resonance Imaging* **20** (4): 319–25. doi:10.1016/S0730-725X(02)00496-4. PMID 12165350.

[21] Laufs, H; Kleinschmidt, A; Beyerle, A; Eger, E; Salek-Haddadi, A; Preibisch, C; Krakow, K (2003). "EEG-correlated fMRI of human alpha activity". *NeuroImage* **19** (4): 1463–76. doi:10.1016/S1053-8119(03)00286-6. PMID 12948703.

[22] Difrancesco, Mark W.; Holland, Scott K.; Szaflarski, Jerzy P. (2008). "Simultaneous EEG/Functional Magnetic Resonance Imaging at 4 Tesla: Correlates of Brain Activity to Spontaneous Alpha Rhythm During Relaxation". *Journal of Clinical Neurophysiology* **25** (5): 255–64. doi:10.1097/WNP.0b013e3181879d56. PMC 2662486. PMID 18791470.

[23] Huizenga, HM; Van Zuijen, TL; Heslenfeld, DJ; Molenaar, PC (2001). "Simultaneous MEG and EEG source analysis". *Physics in medicine and biology* **46** (7): 1737–51. doi:10.1088/0031-9155/46/7/301. PMID 11474922.

[24] Schreckenberger, Mathias; Lange-Asschenfeldt, Christian; Lochmann, Matthias; Mann, Klaus; Siessmeier, Thomas; Buchholz, Hans-Georg; Bartenstein, Peter; Gründer, Gerhard (2004). "The thalamus as the generator and modulator of EEG alpha rhythm: A combined PET/EEG study with lorazepam challenge in humans". *NeuroImage* **22** (2): 637–44. doi:10.1016/j.neuroimage.2004.01.047. PMID 15193592.

[25] The Human Brain in Numbers"The Human Brain in Numbers". *NIH*.

[26] Tatum, W. O., Husain, A. M., Benbadis, S. R. (2008) "Handbook of EEG Interpretation" Demos Medical Publishing.

[27] Nunez PL, Srinivasan R (1981). *Electric fields of the brain: The neurophysics of EEG*. Oxford University Press.

[28] Klein, S.; Thorne, B. M. (3 October 2006). *Biological psychology*. New York, N.Y.: Worth. ISBN 0-7167-9922-7.

[29] Whittingstall, Kevin; Logothetis, Nikos K. (2009). "Frequency-Band Coupling in Surface EEG Reflects Spiking Activity in Monkey Visual Cortex". *Neuron* **64** (2): 281–9. doi:10.1016/j.neuron.2009.08.016. PMID 19874794.

[30] Towle, Vernon L.; Bolaños, José; Suarez, Diane; Tan, Kim; Grzeszczuk, Robert; Levin, David N.; Cakmur, Raif; Frank,

Samuel A.; Spire, Jean-Paul (1993). "The spatial location of EEG electrodes: Locating the best-fitting sphere relative to cortical anatomy". *Electroencephalography and Clinical Neurophysiology* **86** (1): 1–6. doi:10.1016/0013-4694(93)90061-Y. PMID 7678386.

[31] &Na; (1994). "Guideline Seven A Proposal for Standard Montages to Be Used in Clinical EEG". *Journal of Clinical Neurophysiology* **11** (1): 30–6. doi:10.1097/00004691-199401000-00008. PMID 8195424.

[32] Aurlien, H; Gjerde, I.O; Aarseth, J.H; Eldøen, G; Karlsen, B; Skeidsvoll, H; Gilhus, N.E (2004). "EEG background activity described by a large computerized database". *Clinical Neurophysiology* **115** (3): 665–73. doi:10.1016/j.clinph.2003.10.019. PMID 15036063.

[33] Nunez, Paul L.; Pilgreen, Kenneth L. (1991). "The Spline-Laplacian in Clinical Neurophysiology". *Journal of Clinical Neurophysiology* **8** (4): 397–413. doi:10.1097/00004691-199110000-00005. PMID 1761706.

[34] Kondylis, Efstathios D. (2014). "Detection Of High-Frequency Oscillations By Hybrid Depth Electrodes In Standard Clinical Intracranial EEG Recordings.". *Frontiers In Neurology* **5**: 1–10.

[35] Hämäläinen, Matti; Hari, Riitta; Ilmoniemi, Risto J.; Knuutila, Jukka; Lounasmaa, Olli V. (1993). "Magnetoencephalography—theory, instrumentation, and applications to noninvasive studies of the working human brain". *Reviews of Modern Physics* **65** (2): 413–497. Bibcode:1993RvMP...65..413H. doi:10.1103/RevModPhys.65.413.

[36] Murakami, S.; Okada, Y. (13 April 2006). "Contributions of principal neocortical neurons to magnetoencephalography and electroencephalography signals". *The Journal of Physiology* **575** (3): 925–936. doi:10.1113/jphysiol.2006.105379.

[37] Anderson, J. (22 October 2004). *Cognitive Psychology and Its Implications* (Hardcover) (6th ed.). New York, NY: Worth. p. 17. ISBN 0-7167-0110-3.

[38] Creutzfeldt, Otto D; Watanabe, Satoru; Lux, Hans D (1966). "Relations between EEG phenomena and potentials of single cortical cells. I. Evoked responses after thalamic and epicortical stimulation". *Electroencephalography and Clinical Neurophysiology* **20** (1): 1–18. doi:10.1016/0013-4694(66)90136-2. PMID 4161317.

[39] Buzsaki G (2006). *Rhythms of the brain.* Oxford University Press. ISBN 0-19-530106-4.

[40] Tanzer Oguz I. (2006). *Numerical Modeling in Electro- and Magnetoencephalography, Ph.D. Thesis.* Helsinki University of Technology. ISBN 9512280914.

[41] Tatum, William O. (2014). "Ellen R. Grass Lecture: Extraordinary EEG.". *Neurodiagnostic Journal 54.1*: 3–21.

[42] Kirmizi-Alsan, Elif; Bayraktaroglu, Zubeyir; Gurvit, Hakan; Keskin, Yasemin H.; Emre, Murat; Demiralp, Tamer (2006). "Comparative analysis of event-related potentials during Go/NoGo and CPT: Decomposition of electrophysiological markers of response inhibition and sustained attention". *Brain Research* **1104** (1): 114–28. doi:10.1016/j.brainres.2006.03.010. PMID 16824492.

[43] Kisley, Michael A.; Cornwell, Zoe M. (2006). "Gamma and beta neural activity evoked during a sensory gating paradigm: Effects of auditory, somatosensory and cross-modal stimulation". *Clinical Neurophysiology* **117** (11): 2549–63. doi:10.1016/j.clinph.2006.08.003. PMC 1773003. PMID 17008125.

[44] Kanayama, Noriaki; Sato, Atsushi; Ohira, Hideki (2007). "Crossmodal effect with rubber hand illusion and gamma-band activity". *Psychophysiology* **44** (3): 392–402. doi:10.1111/j.1469-8986.2007.00511.x. PMID 17371495.

[45] Gastaut, H (1952). "Electrocorticographic study of the reactivity of rolandic rhythm". *Revue neurologique* **87** (2): 176–82. PMID 13014777.

[46] Oberman, Lindsay M.; Hubbard, Edward M.; McCleery, Joseph P.; Altschuler, Eric L.; Ramachandran, Vilayanur S.; Pineda, Jaime A. (2005). "EEG evidence for mirror neuron dysfunction in autism spectrum disorders". *Cognitive Brain Research* **24** (2): 190–8. doi:10.1016/j.cogbrainres.2005.01.014. PMID 15993757.

[47] Recommendations for the Practice of Clinical Neurophysiology: Guidelines of the International Federation of Clinical Physiology (EEG Suppl. 52) Editors: G. Deuschl and A. Eisen q 1999 International Federation of Clinical Neurophysiology. All rights reserved. Published by Elsevier Science B.V.

[48] Cahn, B. Rael; Polich, John (2006). "Meditation states and traits: EEG, ERP, and neuroimaging studies". *Psychological Bulletin* **132** (2): 180–211. doi:10.1037/0033-2909.132.2.180. PMID 16536641.

[49] Niedermeyer, E (1997). "Alpha rhythms as physiological and abnormal phenomena". *International Journal of Psychophysiology* **26** (1–3): 31–49. doi:10.1016/S0167-8760(97)00754-X. PMID 9202993.

[50] Feshchenko, Vladimir A.; Reinsel, Ruth A.; Veselis, Robert A. (2001). "Multiplicity of the α Rhythm in Normal Humans". *Journal of Clinical Neurophysiology* **18** (4): 331–44. doi:10.1097/00004691-200107000-00005. PMID 11673699.

[51] Pfurtscheller, G.; Lopes Da Silva, F.H. (1999). "Event-related EEG/MEG synchronization and desynchronization: Basic principles". *Clinical Neurophysiology* **110** (11): 1842–57. doi:10.1016/S1388-2457(99)00141-8. PMID 10576479.

[52] Barry, W; Jones, GM (1965). "Influence of Eye Lid Movement Upon Electro-Oculographic Recording of Vertical Eye

Movements". *Aerospace medicine* **36**: 855–8. PMID 14332336.

[53] Iwasaki, Masaki; Kellinghaus, Christoph; Alexopoulos, Andreas V.; Burgess, Richard C.; Kumar, Arun N.; Han, Yanning H.; Lüders, Hans O.; Leigh, R. John (2005). "Effects of eyelid closure, blinks, and eye movements on the electroencephalogram". *Clinical Neurophysiology* **116** (4): 878–85. doi:10.1016/j.clinph.2004.11.001. PMID 15792897.

[54] Lins, Otavio G.; Picton, Terence W.; Berg, Patrick; Scherg, Michael (1993). "Ocular artifacts in EEG and event-related potentials I: Scalp topography". *Brain Topography* **6** (1): 51–63. doi:10.1007/BF01234127. PMID 8260327.

[55] Keren, Alon S.; Yuval-Greenberg, Shlomit; Deouell, Leon Y. (2010). "Saccadic spike potentials in gamma-band EEG: Characterization, detection and suppression". *NeuroImage* **49** (3): 2248–63. doi:10.1016/j.neuroimage.2009.10.057. PMID 19874901.

[56] Yuval-Greenberg, Shlomit; Tomer, Orr; Keren, Alon S.; Nelken, Israel; Deouell, Leon Y. (2008). "Transient Induced Gamma-Band Response in EEG as a Manifestation of Miniature Saccades". *Neuron* **58** (3): 429–41. doi:10.1016/j.neuron.2008.03.027. PMID 18466752.

[57] Epstein, Charles M. (1983). *Introduction to EEG and evoked potentials.* J. B. Lippincot Co. ISBN 0-397-50598-1.

[58] Jung, Tzyy-Ping; Makeig, Scott; Humphries, Colin; Lee, Te-Won; McKeown, Martin J.; Iragui, Vicente; Sejnowski, Terrence J. (2000). "Removing electroencephalographic artifacts by blind source separation". *Psychophysiology* **37** (2): 163–78. doi:10.1017/S0048577200980259. PMID 10731767.

[59] Jung, Tzyy-Ping; Makeig, Scott; Westerfield, Marissa; Townsechesne, Eric; Sejnowski, Terrence J. (2000). "Removal of eye activity artifacts from visual event-related potentials in normal and clinical subjects". *Clinical Neurophysiology* **111** (10): 1745–58. doi:10.1016/S1388-2457(00)00386-2. PMID 11018488.

[60] Joyce, Carrie A.; Gorodnitsky, Irina F.; Kutas, Marta (2004). "Automatic removal of eye movement and blink artifacts from EEG data using blind component separation". *Psychophysiology* **41** (2): 313–25. doi:10.1111/j.1469-8986.2003.00141.x. PMID 15032997.

[61] Fitzgibbon, Sean P; Powers, David M W; Pope, Kenneth J; Clark, C Richard (2007). "Removal of EEG noise and artifact using blind source separation". *Journal of Clinical Neurophysiology* **24** (3): 232–243. doi:10.1097/WNP.0b013e3180556926. PMID 17545826.

[62] Shackman, Alexander J.; McMenamin, Brenton W.; Maxwell, Jeffrey S.; Greischar, Lawrence L.; Davidson, Richard J. (2010). "Identifying robust and sensitive frequency bands for interrogating neural oscillations". *NeuroImage* **51** (4): 1319–33. doi:10.1016/j.neuroimage.2010.03.037. PMC 2871966. PMID 20304076.

[63] Nolan, H.; Whelan, R.; Reilly, R.B. (2010). "FASTER: Fully Automated Statistical Thresholding for EEG artifact Rejection". *Journal of Neuroscience Methods* **192** (1): 152–62. doi:10.1016/j.jneumeth.2010.07.015. PMID 20654646.

[64] Whitham, Emma M; Pope, Kenneth J; Fitzgibbon, Sean P; Lewis, Trent W; Clark, C Richard; Loveless, Stephen; Broberg, Marita; Wallace, Angus; DeLosAngeles, Dylan; Lillie, Peter; et al. (2007). "Scalp electrical recording during paralysis: Quantitative evidence that EEG frequencies above 20Hz are contaminated by EMG". *Clinical neurophysiology* (Elsevier) **118** (8): 1877–1888. doi:10.1016/j.clinph.2007.04.027. PMID 17574912.

[65] Fitzgibbon, Sean P; Lewis, Trent W; Powers, David M W; Whitham, Emma M; Willoughby, John O; Pope, Kenneth J (2013). "Surface Laplacian of Central Scalp Electrical Signals is Insensitive to Muscle Contamination". *IEEE Transactions on Biomedical Engineering* (IEEE) **60** (1): 4–9. doi:10.1109/TBME.2012.2195662. PMID 22542648.

[66] Fitzgibbon, Sean P; DeLosAngeles, Dylan; Lewis, Trent W; Powers, David MW; Whitham, Emma M; Willoughby, John O; Pope, Kenneth J (2014). "Surface Laplacian of scalp electrical signals and independent component analysis resolve EMG contamination of electroencephalogram". *Journal International Journal of Psychophysiology* (Elsevier).

[67] Montez, Teresa; Poil, S.-S.; Jones, B. F.; Manshanden, I.; Verbunt, J. P. A.; Van Dijk, B. W.; Brussaard, A. B.; Van Ooyen, A.; Stam, C. J.; Scheltens, P.; Linkenkaer-Hansen, K. (2009). "Altered temporal correlations in parietal alpha and prefrontal theta oscillations in early-stage Alzheimer disease". *Proceedings of the National Academy of Sciences* **106** (5): 165–70. Bibcode:2009PNAS..106.1614M. doi:10.1073/pnas.0811699106. PMC 2635782. PMID 19164579.

[68] MURI: Synthetic Telepathy. *Cnslab.ss.uci.ed m mm m m* Retrieved 2011-07-19.

[69] "Mind Games". The Economist. 2007-03-23.

[70] Li, Shan (2010-08-08). "Mind reading is on the market". Los Angeles Times.

[71] "Brains-on with NeuroSky and Square Enix's Judecca mind-control game". Engadget. Retrieved 2010-12-02.

[72] "New games powered by brain waves". Physorg.com. Retrieved 2010-12-02.

[73] Snider, Mike (2009-01-07). "Toy trains 'Star Wars' fans to use The Force". *USA Today*. Retrieved 2010-05-01.

[74] "Emotiv Systems Homepage". Emotiv.com. Retrieved 2009-12-29.

[75] "News - NeuroSky Upgrades SDK, Allows For Eye Blink, Brainwave-Powered Games". Gamasutra. 2010-06-30. Retrieved 2010-12-02.

[76] Fiolet, Eliane. "NeuroSky MindWave Brings Brain-Computer Interface to Education". *www.ubergizmo.com*. Ubergizmo.

[77] "NeuroSky MindWave Sets Guinness World Record for "Largest Object Moved Using a Brain-Computer Interface"". *NeuroGadget.com*. NeuroGadget.

[78] http://www.theneurosync.com/

[79] Swartz, Barbara E. (1998). "The advantages of digital over analog recording techniques". *Electroencephalography and Clinical Neurophysiology* **106** (2): 113–7. doi:10.1016/S0013-4694(97)00113-2. PMID 9741771.

[80] Coenen, Anton, Edward Fine, and Oksana Zayachkivska. (2014). "Adolf Beck: A Forgotten Pioneer In Electroencephalography.". *Journal Of The History Of The Neurosciences 23.3*: 276–286.

[81] Pravdich-Neminsky, VV. (1913). "Ein Versuch der Registrierung der elektrischen Gehirnerscheinungen". *Zbl Physiol* **27**: 951–60.

[82] Haas, L F (2003). "Hans Berger (1873-1941), Richard Caton (1842-1926), and electroencephalography". *Journal of Neurology, Neurosurgery & Psychiatry* **74** (1): 9. doi:10.1136/jnnp.74.1.9. PMC 1738204. PMID 12486257.

[83] Millet, David (2002). "The Origins of EEG". *International Society for the History of the Neurosciences* (ISHN).

[84] Keiper, Adam. "The Age of Neuroelectronics". The New Atlantis.

[85] I. Jestrović, J. L. Coyle, E. Sejdić, "Decoding human swallowing via electroencephalography: a state-of-the-art review," Journal of Neural Engineering, vol. 12, no. 5, pp. 051001-1-051001-15, Oct. 2015.

[86] Mind over matter: Brain waves control Asimo 1 Apr 2009, Japan Times

[87] This brain test maps the truth 21 Jul 2008, 0348 hrs IST, Nitasha Natu,TNN

[88] "Puranik, D.A., Joseph, S.K., Daundkar, B.B., Garad, M.V. (2009). Brain Signature profiling in India. Its status as an aid in investigation and as corroborative evidence – as seen from judgments. Proceedings of XX All India Forensic Science Conference, 815 – 822, November 15 – 17, Jaipur." (PDF).

65. Keiper, A. (2006). The age of neuroelectronics. The New Atlantis, 11, 4-41.

2.7.13 Further reading

• Electroencephalogram Paul L. Nunez, Ramesh Srinivasan Scholarpedia 2(2):1348. doi: 10.4249/scholarpedia.1348

2.7.14 External links

• Tanzer Oguz I., (2006) Numerical Modeling in Electro- and Magnetoencephalography, Ph.D. Thesis, Helsinki University of Technology, Finland.

• A tutorial on simulating and estimating EEG sources in Matlab

• A tutorial on analysis of ongoing, evoked, and induced neuronal activity: Power spectra, wavelet analysis, and coherence

• FASTER A fully automated, unsupervised method for processing of high density EEG data. FASTER has been peer-reviewed, it is free and the software is open source. The FASTER software is available here.

• Video demonstration of placement of electrodes

• OpenEEG The OpenEEG project makes hardware plans and software for do-it-yourself EEG devices in an Open Source manner. The hardware is aimed toward amateurs who would like to experiment with EEG.

2.8 Information-theoretic death

The term **Information-theoretic death** relates to physical damage to the brain and the loss of information. It is the destruction of the information within a human brain to such an extent that recovery of the original person is theoretically impossible by any physical means. The concept of information-theoretic death emerged in the 1990s as a response to the progress of medical technology since conditions previously considered as death, such as cardiac arrest, are now reversible, so they can no longer define death.[1] The term alludes to information theory in mathematics.

The term *information-theoretic death* is intended to mean death that is absolutely irreversible by any technology, as distinct from clinical death and legal death, which denote limitations to contextually-available medical care rather than the true theoretical limits of survival. In particular, the prospect of brain repair using molecular nanotechnology raises the possibility that medicine might someday be able to resuscitate patients even hours after the heart stops.

The paper *Molecular Repair of the Brain* by Ralph Merkle defined information-theoretic death as follows:[2]

> A person is dead according to the information-theoretic criterion if their memories, personality, hopes, dreams, etc. have been destroyed in the information-theoretic sense.

That is, if the structures in the brain that encode memory and personality have been so disrupted that it is no longer possible in principle to restore them to an appropriate functional state, then the person is dead. If the structures that encode memory and personality are sufficiently intact that inference of the memory and personality are feasible in principle, and therefore restoration to an appropriate functional state is likewise feasible in principle, then the person is not dead.

The exact timing of information-theoretic death is currently unknown. It has been suggested[3] [4] to occur gradually after many hours of clinical death at room temperature as the brain undergoes autolysis. It may also occur more rapidly if there is no blood flow to the brain during life support, leading to the decomposition stage of brain death, or during the progression of degenerative brain diseases that cause extensive loss of brain structure.

The use of information-theoretic criteria has formed the basis of ethical arguments that state that cryonics is an attempt to save lives rather than being an interment method for the dead. In contrast, if cryonics cannot be applied before information-theoretic death occurs, or if the cryopreservation procedure itself causes information-theoretic death, then cryonics is not feasible. Exactly when complete and total information-theoretic death might occur with respect to different types of preservation and decomposition might also be relevant to the speculative field of mind uploading.

Although the idea of information-theoretic death was first introduced in the context of cryonics,[5] the term has since been used in medical journals discussing issues surrounding brain death[6][7][8] with the same meaning first defined by Merkle.

2.8.1 References

[1] IMR (International Medical Rights)

[2] Merkle, Ralph (January–April 1994), "Molecular Repair of the Brain", *Cryonics*, retrieved 2014-12-27 – via Alcor library online

[3] Merkle, R (1992). "The technical feasibility of cryonics". *Medical Hypotheses* (Elsevier) **39** (1): 6–16. doi:10.1016/0306-9877(92)90133-W. PMID 1435395.

[4] Wowk, B (2014). "The future of death". *Journal of Critical Care* (Elsevier) **29** (6): 1111–1113. doi:10.1016/j.jcrc.2014.08.006. PMID 25194588.

[5] Merkle, R (1992). "The technical feasibility of cryonics". *Medical Hypotheses* (Elsevier) **39** (1): 6–16. doi:10.1016/0306-9877(92)90133-W. PMID 1435395.

[6] Whetstine, L; Streat, S; Darwin, M; Crippen, D (2005). "Pro/con ethics debate: When is dead really dead?". *Critical Care* (BioMed Central) **9** (6): 538–542. doi:10.1186/cc3894. PMID 16356234.

[7] Crippen, DW; Whetstine, L (2007). "Ethics review: Dark angels – the problem of death in intensive care". *Critical Care* (BioMed Central) **11** (1): 202. doi:10.1186/cc5138. PMID 17254317.

[8] Wowk, B (2014). "The future of death". *Journal of Critical Care* (Elsevier) **29** (6): 1111–1113. doi:10.1016/j.jcrc.2014.08.006. PMID 25194588.

2.8.2 External links

- Pro/con ethics debate: When is dead really dead?

- Ethics review: Dark angels-- the problem of death in intensive care

- Albert Einstein's brain and information-theoretic death

- Medical Time Travel by Brian Wowk

2.9 Lazarus sign

The **Lazarus sign** or **Lazarus reflex** is a reflex movement in brain-dead or brainstem failure patients,[1] which causes them to briefly raise their arms and drop them crossed on their chests (in a position similar to some Egyptian mummies).[2][3] The phenomenon is named after the Biblical figure Lazarus of Bethany,[4] whom Jesus is described as having raised from the dead in the Gospel of John.

2.9.1 How it happens

Like the knee jerk reflex, the Lazarus sign is an example of a reflex mediated by a reflex arc – a neural pathway which passes via the spinal column but not through the brain. As a consequence the movement is possible in brain-dead patients whose organs have been kept functioning by life-support machines, precluding the use of complex involuntary motions as a test for brain activity.[3] It has been suggested by neurologists studying the phenomenon that increased awareness of this and similar reflexes "may prevent delays in brain-dead diagnosis and misinterpretations."[2]

The reflex is often preceded by slight shivering motions of the patient's arms, or the appearance of goose bumps on the arms and torso. The arms then begin to flex at the elbows before lifting to be held above the sternum. They are often brought from here towards the neck or chin and touch or cross over. Short exhalations have also been observed coinciding with the action.[3]

2.9.2 Occurrences

The phenomenon has been observed to occur several minutes after the removal of medical ventilators used to pump air in and out of brain-dead patients.[4] It also occurs during testing for apnea – that is, suspension of external breathing and motion of the lung muscles - which is one of the criteria for determining brain death used for example by the American Academy of Neurology.[5]

Occurrences of the Lazarus sign in intensive-care units have been mistaken for evidence of resuscitation of patients. They may frighten those who witness the movement, and have been viewed by some as miraculous events.[3] [4]

2.9.3 See also

- Lazarus syndrome

2.9.4 References

[1] "Brain death and brainstem failure". The Egyptian Society of Medical Ethics. 2009. Retrieved August 26, 2011.

[2] S.G Han et. al (2006). "Reflex Movements in Patients with Brain Death: A Prospective Study in A Tertiary Medical Center". *Journal of Korean medical science* **21** (3): 588–90. doi:10.3346/jkms.2006.21.3.588. ISSN 1011-8934. PMC 2729975. PMID 16778413.

[3] Allan H Ropper (1984). "Unusual spontaneous movements in brain-dead patients". *Neurology* **34** (8): 1089–90. doi:10.1212/wnl.34.8.1089. PMID 6540387.

[4] Calixto Machado (2007). *Brain death: a reappraisal.* Springer. p. 79. ISBN 978-0-387-38975-2.

[5] "Practice Parameters: Determining Brain Death in Adults" (PDF). American Academy of Neurology. 1994. Retrieved 12 July 2009.

2.10 Legal death

Legal death is a government's official recognition that a person has died. Normally this is done by issuing a death certificate. In most cases, such a certificate is only issued either by a doctor's declaration of death or by an identified corpse.

2.10.1 Medical declaration

See also: Medical definition of death

In hospitals or other care facilities, a doctor or other qualified person legally declares a person dead. Medical advances have made death more difficult to define.

2.10.2 Presumption of death

Main article: Declared death in absentia

In some cases, a person will be declared dead even without any remains or doctor's declaration. This is under one of two circumstances. First, if a person was known to be in mortal peril when last seen, they can often be declared dead shortly after. Examples would be the passengers of the *Titanic* that were not rescued after the ship sank. Second, if a person has not been seen for a certain period of time and there has been no evidence that they are alive. The amount of time that has passed varies by jurisdiction, from as little as four years in the US state of Georgia to twenty years in Italy.

2.10.3 Fraudulent death

In some cases, a legal declaration of death is fraudulent. Several people have faked their own deaths for various reasons. The most common reasons for this are to collect insurance money, to avoid capture by police or to avoid paying debts.

People have also been declared legally dead by corrupt governments. In Uttar Pradesh, India, officials have often been bribed to declare a living person legally dead so that others can steal their land or other property. The Uttar Pradesh Association of Dead People was founded to help people in this situation.

2.10.4 Investigation

Determining cause of death often has important legal implications. Governments appoint a coroner to both determine cause of death, and if necessary, identify bodies when their identities are unknown. Deaths are usually classified as natural, accidental, homicide or suicide. A soldier is often listed as killed in action if the death was during military service. There are legal implications to all of the classifications.

2.10.5   Estate

Main article: Probate

In nearly all jurisdictions, dead people do not have the right to own property. When a person dies, their property needs to be distributed to others in a process called probate. People can specify their wishes before they die by preparing a will and testament. If there is no will, the laws of their country determine how the property is distributed. In most cases, it would go to next of kin, such as a spouse or adult child. If the person who died is wealthy, often a portion of their property will be collected by an estate tax.

2.10.6   Reversal

In some cases, declarations of death are in error and need to be reversed. One such example is after an erroneous declaration of death. Another is for fraud. In some jurisdictions, a declaration of death is final and nearly impossible to reverse. In most places, it is a long drawn-out process. It took Lal Bihari nineteen years to reverse his fraudulent legal death.

2.10.7   References

- Uniform Determination of Death Act – Uniform Law Commission

2.11   Life support

Life support refers to the treatments and techniques performed in an emergency in order to support life after the failure of one or more vital organs. Healthcare providers and emergency medical technicians are generally certified to perform basic and advanced life support procedures; however, basic life support is sometimes provided at the scene of an emergency by family members or bystanders before emergency services arrive. In the case of cardiac injuries, cardiopulmonary resuscitation is initiated by bystanders or family members 25% of the time. Basic life support techniques, such as performing CPR on a victim of cardiac arrest, can double or even triple that patient's chance of survival.[1] Other types of basic life support include relief from choking, staunching of bleeding, first aid, and the use of an automated external defibrillator.

The purpose of basic life support (abbreviated BLS) is to save lives in a variety of different situations that require immediate attention. These situations can include, but

are not limited to, cardiac arrest, stroke, drowning, choking, accidental injuries, violence, severe allergic reactions, burns, hypothermia, birth complications, drug overdose, and alcohol intoxication. The most common emergency that requires BLS is cerebral hypoxia, a shortage of oxygen to the brain due to heart or respiratory failure. A victim of cerebral hypoxia may die within 8–10 minutes without basic life support procedures. BLS is the lowest level of emergency care, followed by advanced life support and critical care.[2]

2.11.1   Bioethics

As technology continues to advance within the medical field, so do the options available for healthcare. Out of respect for the patient's autonomy, patients and their families are able to make their own decisions about life-sustaining treatment or whether to hasten death.[3] When patients and their families are forced to make decisions concerning life support as a form of end-of-life or emergency treatment, ethical dilemmas often arise. When a patient is terminally ill or seriously injured, medical interventions can save or prolong the life of the patient. Because such treatment is available, families are often faced with the moral question of whether or not to treat the patient. Between 60 and 70% of seriously ill patients will not be able to decide for themselves whether or not they want to limit treatments, including life support measures. This leaves these difficult decisions up to loved ones and family members.

Patients and family members who wish to limit the treatment provided to the patient may complete a do not resuscitate (DNR) or do not intubate (DNI) order with their doctor. These orders state that the patient does not wish to receive these forms of life support. Generally, DNRs and DNIs are justified for patients who might not benefit from CPR, who would result in permanent damage from CPR or patients who have a poor quality of life prior to CPR or intubation and do not wish to prolong the dying process.

Another type of life support that presents ethical arguments is the placement of a feeding tube. Decisions about hydration and nutrition are generally the most ethically challenging when it comes to end-of-life care. In 1990, the US Supreme Court ruled that artificial nutrition and hydration are not different from other life-supporting treatments. Because of this, artificial nutrition and hydration can be refused by a patient or their family. A person cannot live without food and water, and because of this, it has been argued that withholding food and water is similar to the act of killing the patient or even allowing the person to die.[4] This type of voluntary death is referred to as passive euthanasia.[5]

2.11.2   Techniques

There are many therapies and techniques that may be used by clinicians to achieve the goal of sustaining life. Some examples include:

- Feeding tube

- Total parenteral nutrition

- Mechanical ventilation

- Heart/Lung bypass

- Urinary catheterization

- Dialysis

- Cardiopulmonary resuscitation

- Defibrillation

- Artificial pacemaker

- Life extension

- Life support system for human spaceflight.[6]

These techniques are applied most commonly in the Emergency Department, Intensive Care Unit and, Operating Rooms. As various life support technologies have improved and evolved they are used increasingly outside of the hospital environment. For example, a patient who requires a ventilator for survival is commonly discharged home with these devices. Another example includes the now-ubiquitous presence of automated external defibrillators in public venues which allow lay people to deliver life support in a prehospital environment.

The ultimate goals of life support depend on the specific patient situation. Typically, life support is used to sustain life while the underlying injury or illness is being treated or evaluated for prognosis. Life support techniques may also be used indefinitely if the underlying medical condition cannot be corrected, but a reasonable quality of life can still be expected.

2.11.3   Gallery

- Dialysis center for patients with severe chronic kidney disease

- Hemodialysis machine Bellco Formula

- Endotracheal tube of an emergency ventilator system

- An iron lung

- Ventilator "Evita4" on an ICU

2.11.4   References

[1] What is CPR [Internet]. 2013. American heart association; [cited 2013 Nov 5]. Available from: http://www.heart.org/ HEARTORG/CPRAndECC/WhatisCPR/What-is-CPR_ UCM_001120_SubHomePage.jsp

[2] Alic M. 2013. Basic life support (BLS) [Internet]. 3rd. Detroit (MI):Gale ; [2013, cited 2013 Nov 5] Available from: http://go.galegroup. com/ps/i.do?id=GALE%7CCX2760400129&v=2. 1&u=csumb_main&it=r&p=GVRL&sw=w&asid= 40d96ff26746d55939f14dbf57297410

[3] Beauchamp, Tom L., LeRoy Walters, Jefferey P. Kahn, and Anna C. Mastroianni. "Death and Dying." Contemporary Issues in Bioethics. Wadsworth: Cengage Learning, 2008. 397. Web. 9 Nov. 2013.

[4] Abbot-Penny A, Bartels P, Paul B, Rawles L, Ward A [2005]. End of Life Care: An Ethical Overview. Ethical Challenges in End of Life Care. [Internet]. [cited 2013 Nov 6]. Available from: www.ahc.umn.edu/img/assets/26104/ End_of_Life.pdf life support bioethics

[5] Beauchamp, Tom L., LeRoy Walters, Jefferey P. Kahn, and Anna C. Mastroianni. "Death and Dying." Contemporary Issues in Bioethics. Wadsworth: Cengage Learning, 2008. 402. Web. 9 Nov. 2013.

[6] "International Space Station Environmental Control and Life Support System" (PDF). NASA. Retrieved 11 December 2010.

2.12   Locked-in syndrome

Locked-in syndrome (**LIS**) is a condition in which a patient is aware but cannot move or communicate verbally due to complete paralysis of nearly all voluntary muscles in the body except for the eyes. **Total locked-in syndrome** is a version of locked-in syndrome wherein the eyes are paralyzed as well.[1] Fred Plum and Jerome Posner coined the term for this disorder in 1966.[2][3] Locked-in syndrome is also known as **cerebromedullospinal disconnection**,[4] **de-efferented state**, **pseudocoma**,[5] and **ventral pontine syndrome**.

2.12.1   Presentation

Locked-in syndrome usually results in quadriplegia and the inability to speak in otherwise cognitively intact individuals. Those with locked-in syndrome may be able to communicate with others through coded messages by blinking or moving their eyes, which are often not affected by the paralysis. The symptoms are similar to those of sleep paralysis. Patients who have locked-in syndrome are conscious and aware, with no loss of cognitive function. They can sometimes retain proprioception and sensation throughout their bodies. Some patients may have the ability to move certain facial muscles, and most often some or all of the extraocular eye muscles. Individuals with the syndrome lack coordination between breathing and voice.[6] This restricts them from producing voluntary sounds, though the vocal cords are not paralysed.[6]

2.12.2 Causes

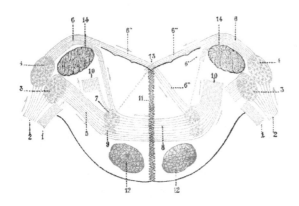

In children, the most common cause is a stroke of the ventral pons.[7]

Unlike persistent vegetative state, in which the upper portions of the brain are damaged and the lower portions are spared, locked-in syndrome is caused by damage to specific portions of the lower brain and brainstem, with no damage to the upper brain.

Possible causes of locked-in syndrome include:

- Snakebite cases - More frequently from a krait bite and other neurotoxic venoms, as they cannot, usually, cross the blood–brain barrier

- Amyotrophic lateral sclerosis (aka Lou Gehrig's disease)

- Brainstem stroke

- Diseases of the circulatory system

- Medication overdose , or central pontine myelinolysis secondary to rapid correction of hyponatremia

- Multiple sclerosis

- Damage to nerve cells, particularly destruction of the myelin sheath, caused by disease or central pontine myelinolysis secondary to rapid correction of hyponatremia [>1 mEq/L/h])

- A stroke or brain hemorrhage, usually of the basilar artery

- Traumatic brain injury

2.12.3 Diagnosis

Curare poisoning mimics a total locked-in syndrome by causing paralysis of all voluntarily controlled skeletal muscles.[8] The respiratory muscles are also paralyzed, but the victim can be kept alive by artificial respiration, such as mouth-to-mouth resuscitation. In a study of 29 army volunteers who were paralyzed with curare, artificial respiration managed to keep an oxygen saturation of always above 85%,[9] a level at which there is no evidence of altered state of consciousness.[10] Spontaneous breathing is resumed after the end of the duration of action of curare, which is generally between 30 minutes[11] and eight hours,[12] depending on the variant of the toxin and dosage.

2.12.4 Treatment

Neither a standard treatment nor a cure is available. Stimulation of muscle reflexes with electrodes (NMES) has been known to help patients regain some muscle function. Other courses of treatment are often symptomatic.[13] Assistive computer interface technologies, such as Dasher, or OptiKey, combined with eye tracking, may be used to help patients communicate.

2.12.5 Prognosis

Extremely rarely does any significant motor function return. The majority of locked-in syndrome patients do not regain motor control, but devices are available to help patients communicate. Within the first four months after its onset, 90% of those with this condition die. However, some people with the condition continue to live much longer,[14][15] while in exceptional cases, like that of Kerry Pink[16] and Kate Allatt,[17] a full spontaneous recovery may be achieved.

2.12.6 Research

New direct brain interface mechanisms may provide future remedies; one effort in 2002 allowed a fully locked-in patient to answer yes-or-no questions.[18][19][20] Some scientists have reported that they have developed a technique that allows locked-in patients to communicate via sniffing.[21]

2.12.7 See also

- Akinetic mutism

- Brain death

- Martin Pistorius, author who wrote autobiographical *Ghost Boy*

- The Diving Bell and the Butterfly

- The Diving Bell and the Butterfly (film)

2.12.8   References

[1] Bauer, G. and Gerstenbrand, F. and Rumpl, E. (1979). "Varieties of the locked-in syndrome". *Journal of Neurology* **221** (2): 77–91. doi:10.1007/BF00313105. PMID 92545.

[2] Agranoff, Adam B. "Stroke Motor Impairment". *eMedicine*. Retrieved 2007-11-29.

[3] Plum, F; Posner, JB (1966), *The diagnosis of stupor and coma*, Philadelphia, PA, USA: FA Davis, 197 pp.

[4] Nordgren RE, Markesbery WR, Fukuda K, Reeves AG (1971). "Seven cases of cerebromedullospinal disconnection: the "locked-in" syndrome". *Neurology* **21** (11): 1140–8. doi:10.1212/wnl.21.11.1140. PMID 5166219.

[5] Flügel KA, Fuchs HH, Druschky KF (1977). "The "locked-in" syndrome: pseudocoma in thrombosis of the basilar artery (author's trans.)". *Dtsch. Med. Wochenschr.* (in German) **102** (13): 465–70. doi:10.1055/s-0028-1104912. PMID 844425.

[6] Fager, Susan; Beukelman, Karantounis, Jakobs (2006). "Use of safe-laser access technology to increase head movements in persons with severe motor impairments: a series of case reports". *Augmentative and Alternative Communication* **22** (3): 222–29. doi:10.1080/07434610600650318. PMID 17114165.

[7] Bruno MA, Schnakers C, Damas F, et al. (October 2009). "Locked-in syndrome in children: report of five cases and review of the literature". *Pediatr. Neurol.* **41** (4): 237–46. doi:10.1016/j.pediatrneurol.2009.05.001. PMID 19748042.

[8] Page 357 in: Damasio, Antonio R. (1999). *The feeling of what happens: body and emotion in the making of consciousness*. San Diego: Harcourt Brace. ISBN 0-15-601075-5.

[9] Page 520 in: Paradis, Norman A. (2007). *Cardiac arrest: the science and practice of resuscitation medicine*. Cambridge, UK: Cambridge University Press. ISBN 0-521-84700-1.

[10] Oxymoron: Our Love-Hate Relationship with Oxygen, By Mike McEvoy at Albany Medical College, New York. 10/12/2010

[11] For therapeutic dose of tubocurarine by shorter limit as given at page 151 in: Rang, H. P. (2003). *Pharmacology*. Edinburgh: Churchill Livingstone. ISBN 0-443-07145-4. OCLC 51622037.

[12] For 20-fold paralytic dose of toxiferine ("calebas curare"), according to: Page 330 in: *The Alkaloids: v. 1: A Review of Chemical Literature (Specialist Periodical Reports)*. Cambridge, Eng: Royal Society of Chemistry. 1971. ISBN 0-85186-257-8.

[13] *lockedinsyndrome* at NINDS

[14] Joshua Foer (October 2, 2008). "The Unspeakable Odyssey of the Motionless Boy". *Esquire*.

[15] Piotr Kniecicki "An art of graceful dying". Clitheroe: Łukasz Świderski, 2014, s. 73. ISBN 978-0-9928486-0-6

[16] Stephen Nolan (August 16, 2010). "I recovered from locked-in syndrome". *BBC Radio 5 Live*.

[17] "Woman's recovery from 'locked-in' syndrome". *BBC News*. March 14, 2012.

[18] Parker, I., "Reading Minds," The New Yorker, January 20, 2003, 52–63

[19] Berdik, Chris (October 15, 2008), "Turning Thoughts into Words", *BU Today* (Research), Boston University.

[20] Keiper, Adam (Winter 2006). "The Age of Neuroelectronics". The New Atlantis. pp. 4–41.

[21] "'Locked-In' Patients Can Follow Their Noses". Science Mag. 26 Jul 2010. Retrieved 27 Jul 2010.

2.12.9   Further reading

- Piotr Kniecicki (2014). *An Art of Graceful Dying*. Lukasz Swiderski ISBN 978-0-9928486-0-6 (Autobiography, written while residual wrist movements and specially adapted computer.)

2.12.10   External links

- The Unlock Project

- Locked-In Syndrome Association's guide to communicating without language (French)

- Rachel's Communication boards – for when you need to communicate with someone with LIS.

- OptiKey .

2.13   Mechanical ventilation

For the use in architecture and climate control, see Ventilation (architecture).

In medicine, **mechanical ventilation** is a method to mechanically assist or replace spontaneous breathing. This may involve a machine called a ventilator or the breathing may be assisted by a registered nurse, physician, physician assistant, respiratory therapist, paramedic, or other suitable person compressing a bag or set of bellows. Mechanical ventilation is termed "invasive" if it involves any instrument penetrating through the mouth (such as an endotracheal tube) or the skin (such as a tracheostomy tube).[1] There are two main modes of mechanical ventilation within the two divisions: positive pressure ventilation, where air (or another gas mix) is pushed into the trachea, and negative pressure ventilation, where air is, in essence, sucked into the lungs.

2.13.1   Medical uses

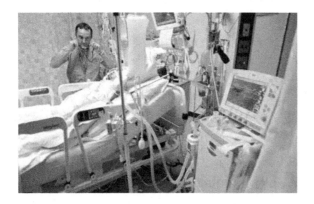

Respiratory therapist examining a mechanically ventilated patient on an Intensive Care Unit.

Mechanical ventilation is indicated when the patient's spontaneous ventilation is inadequate to maintain life. It is also indicated as prophylaxis for imminent collapse of other physiologic functions, or ineffective gas exchange in the lungs. Because mechanical ventilation serves only to provide assistance for breathing and does not cure a disease, the patient's underlying condition should be correctable and should resolve over time. In addition, other factors must be taken into consideration because mechanical ventilation is not without its complications (see below)

Common medical indications for use include:

- Acute lung injury (including ARDS, trauma)

- Apnea with respiratory arrest, including cases from intoxication

- Acute severe asthma, requiring intubation

- Chronic obstructive pulmonary disease (COPD)

- Acute respiratory acidosis with partial pressure of carbon dioxide (pCO_2) > 50 mmHg and pH < 7.25, which may be due to paralysis of the diaphragm due to Guillain-Barré syndrome, myasthenia gravis, motor neuron disease, spinal cord injury, or the effect of anaesthetic and muscle relaxant drugs

- Increased work of breathing as evidenced by significant tachypnea, retractions, and other physical signs of respiratory distress

- Hypoxemia with arterial partial pressure of oxygen (PaO_2) < 55 mm Hg with supplemental fraction of inspired oxygen (FiO_2) = 1.0

- Hypotension including sepsis, shock, congestive heart failure

- Neurological diseases such as muscular dystrophy and amyotrophic lateral sclerosis

2.13.2   Associated risk

Barotrauma — Pulmonary barotrauma is a well-known complication of positive-pressure mechanical ventilation.[2] This includes pneumothorax, subcutaneous emphysema, pneumomediastinum, and pneumoperitoneum.[2]

Ventilator-associated lung injury — Ventilator-associated lung injury (VALI) refers to acute lung injury that occurs during mechanical ventilation. It is clinically indistinguishable from acute lung injury or acute respiratory distress syndrome (ALI/ARDS).[3]

Diaphragm — Controlled mechanical ventilation may lead to a rapid type of disuse atrophy involving the diaphragmatic muscle fibers, which can develop within the first day of mechanical ventilation.[4] This cause of atrophy in the diaphragm is also a cause of atrophy in all respiratory related muscles during controlled mechanical ventilation.[5]

Motility of mucocilia in the airways — Positive pressure ventilation appears to impair mucociliary motility in the airways. Bronchial mucus transport was frequently impaired and associated with retention of secretions and pneumonia.[6]

Complications

Mechanical ventilation is often a life-saving intervention, but carries potential complications including pneumothorax, airway injury, alveolar damage, and ventilator-associated pneumonia.[7] Other complications include diaphragm atrophy, decreased cardiac output, and oxygen toxicity. One of the primary complications that presents in patients mechanically ventilated is acute lung injury (ALI)/acute respiratory distress syndrome (ARDS). ALI/ARDS are recognized as significant contributors to patient morbidity and mortality.[8]

In many healthcare systems, prolonged ventilation as part of intensive care is a limited resource (in that there are only so many patients that can receive care at any given moment). It is used to support a single failing organ system (the lungs) and cannot reverse any underlying disease process (such as terminal cancer). For this reason, there can be (occasionally difficult) decisions to be made about whether it is suitable to commence someone on mechanical ventilation. Equally many ethical issues surround the decision to discontinue mechanical ventilation.[9]

2.13.3 Application and duration

It can be used as a short-term measure, for example during an operation or critical illness (often in the setting of an intensive-care unit). It may be used at home or in a nursing or rehabilitation institution if patients have chronic illnesses that require long-term ventilatory assistance. Due to the anatomy of the human pharynx, larynx, and esophagus and the circumstances for which ventilation is needed, additional measures are often required to secure the airway during positive-pressure ventilation in order to allow unimpeded passage of air into the trachea and avoid air passing into the esophagus and stomach. The common method is by insertion of a tube into the trachea: intubation, which provides a clear route for the air. This can be either an endotracheal tube, inserted through the natural openings of mouth or nose, or a tracheostomy inserted through an artificial opening in the neck. In other circumstances simple airway maneuvres, an oropharyngeal airway or laryngeal mask airway may be employed. If the patient is able to protect his/her own airway and non-invasive ventilation or negative-pressure ventilation is used then an airway adjunct may not be needed.

Negative pressure machines

Main article: Negative pressure ventilator

The iron lung, also known as the Drinker and Shaw tank, was developed in 1929 and was one of the first negative-pressure machines used for long-term ventilation. It was refined and used in the 20th century largely as a result of the polio epidemic that struck the world in the 1940s. The machine is, in effect, a large elongated tank, which encases the patient up to the neck. The neck is sealed with a rubber

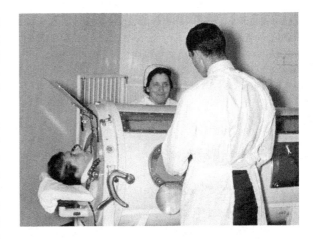

An iron lung

gasket so that the patient's face (and airway) are exposed to the room air.

While the exchange of oxygen and carbon dioxide between the bloodstream and the pulmonary airspace works by diffusion and requires no external work, air must be moved into and out of the lungs to make it available to the gas exchange process. In spontaneous breathing, a negative pressure is created in the pleural cavity by the muscles of respiration, and the resulting gradient between the atmospheric pressure and the pressure inside the thorax generates a flow of air.

In the iron lung by means of a pump, the air is withdrawn mechanically to produce a vacuum inside the tank, thus creating negative pressure. This negative pressure leads to expansion of the chest, which causes a decrease in intrapulmonary pressure, and increases flow of ambient air into the lungs. As the vacuum is released, the pressure inside the tank equalizes to that of the ambient pressure, and the elastic coil of the chest and lungs leads to passive exhalation. However, when the vacuum is created, the abdomen also expands along with the lung, cutting off venous flow back to the heart, leading to pooling of venous blood in the lower extremities. There are large portholes for nurse or home assistant access. The patients can talk and eat normally, and can see the world through a well-placed series of mirrors. Some could remain in these iron lungs for years at a time quite successfully.

Today, negative pressure mechanical ventilators are still in use, notably with the polio wing hospitals in England such as St Thomas' Hospital in London and the John Radcliffe in Oxford. The prominent device used is a smaller device known as the cuirass. The cuirass is a shell-like unit, creating negative pressure only to the chest using a combination of a fitting shell and a soft bladder. Its main use is in patients with neuromuscular disorders that have some residual muscular function. However, it was prone to falling off and caused severe chafing and skin damage and was not used as a long-term device. In recent years this device has re-surfaced as a modern polycarbonate shell with multiple seals and a high-pressure oscillation pump in order to carry out biphasic cuirass ventilation.

Positive pressure

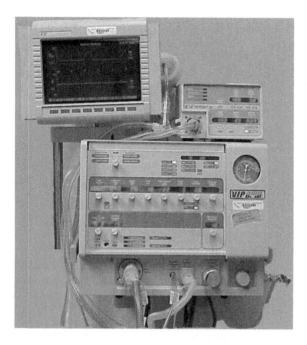

Neonatal mechanical ventilator

The design of the modern positive-pressure ventilators were based mainly on technical developments by the military during World War II to supply oxygen to fighter pilots in high altitude. Such ventilators replaced the iron lungs as safe endotracheal tubes with high-volume/low-pressure cuffs were developed. The popularity of positive-pressure ventilators rose during the polio epidemic in the 1950s in Scandinavia and the United States and was the beginning of modern ventilation therapy. Positive pressure through manual supply of 50% oxygen through a tracheostomy tube led to a reduced mortality rate among patients with polio and respiratory paralysis. However, because of the sheer amount of man-power required for such manual intervention, mechanical positive-pressure ventilators became increasingly popular.

Positive-pressure ventilators work by increasing the patient's airway pressure through an endotracheal or tracheostomy tube. The positive pressure allows air to flow into the airway until the ventilator breath is terminated. Then, the airway pressure drops to zero, and the elastic recoil of the chest wall and lungs push the tidal volume — the breath-out through passive exhalation.

Transairway pressure

$$P_{TA} = (P_{AO}) - (P_{ALV})$$

- PTA =Transairway pressure
- PAO = Pressure at airway opening
- PALV = Pressure in alveoli

2.13.4   Types of ventilators

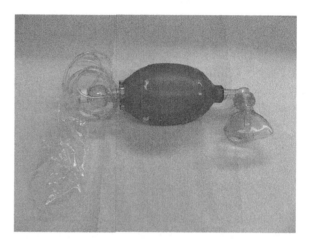

SMART BAG MO Bag-Valve-Mask Resuscitator

Ventilators come in many different styles and method of giving a breath to sustain life. There are manual ventilators such as bag valve masks and anesthesia bags that require the users to hold the ventilator to the face or to an artificial airway and maintain breaths with their hands. Mechanical ventilators are ventilators not requiring operator effort and are typically computer-controlled or pneumatic-controlled.

Mechanical ventilators

Mechanical ventilators typically require power by a battery or a wall outlet (DC or AC) though some ventilators work on a pneumatic system not requiring power.

- **Transport ventilators** — These ventilators are small and more rugged, and can be powered pneumatically or via AC or DC power sources.

- **Intensive-care ventilators** — These ventilators are larger and usually run on AC power (though virtually all contain a battery to facilitate intra-facility transport and as a back-up in the event of a power failure). This style of ventilator often provides greater control of a wide variety of ventilation parameters (such as inspiratory rise time). Many ICU ventilators also incorporate graphics to provide visual feedback of each breath.

- **Neonatal ventilators** — Designed with the preterm neonate in mind, these are a specialized subset of ICU ventilators that are designed to deliver the smaller, more precise volumes and pressures required to ventilate these patients.

- **Positive airway pressure ventilators (PAP)** — These ventilators are specifically designed for non-invasive ventilation. This includes ventilators for use at home for treatment of chronic conditions such as sleep apnea or COPD.

2.13.5 Breath delivery

Trigger

The trigger is what causes a breath to be delivered by a mechanical ventilator. Breaths may be triggered by a patient taking their own breath, a ventilator operator pressing a manual breath button, or by the ventilator based on the set breath rate and mode of ventilation.

Cycle

The cycle is what causes the breath to transition from the inspiratory phase to the exhalation phase. Breaths may be cycled by a mechanical ventilator when a set time has been reached, or when a preset flow or percentage of the maximum flow delivered during a breath is reached depending on the breath type and the settings. Breaths can also be cycled when an alarm condition such as a high pressure limit has been reached, which is a primary strategy in pressure regulated volume control.

Limit

Limit is how the breath is controlled. Breaths may be limited to a set maximum circuit pressure or a set maximum flow.

2.13.6 Breath exhalation

Exhalation in mechanical ventilation is almost always completely passive. The ventilator's expiratory valve is opened, and expiratory flow is allowed until the baseline pressure (PEEP) is reached. Expiratory flow is determined by patient factors such as compliance and resistance.

2.13.7 Dead space

Mechanical dead space is defined as the volume of gas rebreathed as the result of use in a mechanical device.

Example of calculation for mechanical dead space

$$V_{Dmech} = V_T - V_{Dphys} - \frac{PaCO2(V_T - V_D - V_{Dmech})}{P_{ACO_2}}$$

Simplified version

$$\frac{V_D}{V_T} = \frac{PaCO_2 - P\bar{E}CO_2}{PaCO_2}$$

2.13.8 Modes of ventilation

Main article: Modes of mechanical ventilation

Mechanical ventilation utilizes several separate systems for ventilation referred to as the mode. Modes come in many different delivery concepts but all modes fall into one of three categories; volume-cycled, pressure-cycled, spontaneously cycled. In general, the selection of which mode of mechanical ventilation to use for a given patient is based on the familiarity of clinicians with modes and the equipment availability at a particular institution.[10]

2.13.9 Modification of settings

In adults when 100% Oxygen (O2) (1.00 *FiO*2) is used initially, it is easy to calculate the next *FiO*2 to be used and easy to estimate the shunt fraction. The estimated shunt fraction refers to the amount of oxygen not being absorbed into the circulation. In normal physiology, gas exchange (oxygen/carbon dioxide) occurs at the level of the alveoli in the lungs. The existence of a shunt refers to any process that hinders this gas exchange, leading to wasted oxygen inspired and the flow of un-oxygenated blood back to the left heart (which ultimately supplies the rest of the body with unoxygenated blood).

When using 100% O2 (*FiO*2 1.00), the degree of shunting is estimated by subtracting the measured *PaO*2 (from an arterial blood gas) from 700 mmHg. For each difference of 100 mmHg, the shunt is 5%. A shunt of more than 25% should prompt a search for the cause of this hypoxemia, such as mainstem intubation or pneumothorax, and should be treated accordingly. If such complications are not present, other causes must be sought after, and positive end-expiratory pressure (PEEP) should be used to treat this intrapulmonary shunt. Other such causes of a shunt include:

- Alveolar collapse from major atelectasis

- Alveolar collection of material other than gas, such as pus from pneumonia, water and protein from acute respiratory distress syndrome, water from congestive heart failure, or blood from haemorrhage

Weaning from mechanical ventilation

Withdrawal from mechanical ventilation—also known as weaning—should not be delayed unnecessarily, nor should it be done prematurely. Patients should have their ventilation considered for withdrawal if they are able to support their own ventilation and oxygenation, and this should be assessed continuously. There are several objective parameters to look for when considering withdrawal, but there are no specific criteria that generalizes to all patients.

The Rapid Shallow Breathing Index (RSBI, the ratio of respiratory frequency to tidal volume (f/VT), previously referred to as the "Tobin Index" after Dr. Martin Tobin of Loyola University Medical Center) is one of the best studied and most commonly used weaning predictors, with no other predictor having been shown to be superior. It was described in a prospective cohort study of mechanically ventilated patients which found that a RSBI > 105 breaths/min/L was associated with weaning failure, while a RSBI < 105 breaths/min/L predicted weaning success with a sensitivity, specificity, positive predictive value and negative predictive value of 97%, 64%, 78%, 95% respectively.[11]

2.13.10   Respiratory monitoring

Main article: respiratory monitoring
 One of the main reasons why a patient is admitted to an

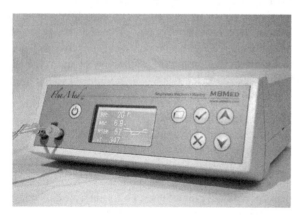

Respiratory mechanics monitor

ICU is for delivery of mechanical ventilation. Monitoring a patient in mechanical ventilation has many clinical applications: Enhance understanding of pathophysiology, aid with

diagnosis, guide patient management, avoid complications and assessment of trends.[12]

Most of modern ventilators have basic monitoring tools. There are also monitors that work independently of the ventilator, which allow to measure patients after the ventilator has been removed, such as a T tube test.

2.13.11   Artificial airways as a connection to the ventilator

Main article: Artificial airway

There are various procedures and mechanical devices that provide protection against airway collapse, air leakage, and aspiration:

- Face mask — In resuscitation and for minor procedures under anaesthesia, a face mask is often sufficient to achieve a seal against air leakage. Airway patency of the unconscious patient is maintained either by manipulation of the jaw or by the use of *nasopharyngeal* or *oropharyngeal airway*. These are designed to provide a passage of air to the pharynx through the nose or mouth, respectively. Poorly fitted masks often cause nasal bridge ulcers, a problem for some patients. Face masks are also used for non-invasive ventilation in conscious patients. A full face mask does not, however, provide protection against aspiration.

- *Tracheal intubation* is often performed for mechanical ventilation of hours to weeks duration. A tube is inserted through the nose (nasotracheal intubation) or mouth (orotracheal intubation) and advanced into the trachea. In most cases, tubes with inflatable cuffs are used for protection against leakage and aspiration. Intubation with a cuffed tube is thought to provide the best protection against aspiration. Tracheal tubes inevitably cause pain and coughing. Therefore, unless a patient is unconscious or anaesthetized for other reasons, sedative drugs are usually given to provide tolerance of the tube. Other disadvantages of tracheal intubation include damage to the mucosal lining of the nasopharynx or oropharynx and subglottic stenosis.

- *Supraglottic airway* — a supraglottic airway (SGA) is any airway device that is seated above and outside the trachea, as an alternative to endotracheal intubation. Most devices work via masks or cuffs that inflate to isolate the trachea for oxygen delivery. Newer devices feature esophageal ports for suctioning or ports for tube exchange to allow intubation. Supraglottic airways differ primarily from tracheal intubation in that they do not prevent aspiration. After the introduction of the laryngeal mask airway (LMA) in 1998, supraglottic airway devices have become mainstream in both elective and emergency anesthesia.[13] There are many types of SGAs available including the Esophageal-tracheal Combitube (ETC), Laryngeal tube (LT), and the obsolete Esophageal obturator airway (EOA).

- *Cricothyrotomy* — Patients requiring emergency airway management, in whom tracheal intubation has been unsuccessful, may require an airway inserted through a surgical opening in the cricothyroid membrane. This is similar to a tracheostomy but a cricothyrotomy is reserved for emergency access.[14]

- *Tracheostomy* — When patients require mechanical ventilation for several weeks, a tracheostomy may provide the most suitable access to the trachea. A tracheostomy is a surgically created passage into the trachea. Tracheostomy tubes are well-tolerated and often do not necessitate any use of sedative drugs. Tracheostomy tubes may be inserted early during treatment in patients with pre-existing severe respiratory disease, or in any patient expected to be difficult to wean from mechanical ventilation, i.e., patients with little muscular reserve.

- *Mouthpiece* — Less common interface, does not provide protection against aspiration. There are lipseal mouthpieces with flanges to help hold them in place if patient is unable.

2.13.12 Ventilation formulas

Alveolar Ventilation

$$\dot{V}_A = (V_T - V_{DSphys}) \times f$$

Arterial PaCO2

$$PaCO_2 = \frac{0.863 \times \dot{V}_{CO_2}}{\dot{V}_A}$$

Alveolar volume

$$V_A = V_T - V_f$$

Estimated physiologic shunt equation

$$\frac{Q_{SP}}{Q_T} = \frac{CcO_2 - CaO_2}{5 + (CcO_2 - CaO_2)}$$

2.13.13 History

The Roman physician Galen may have been the first to describe mechanical ventilation: "If you take a dead animal and blow air through its larynx [through a reed], you will fill its bronchi and watch its lungs attain the greatest distention."[15] Vesalius too describes ventilation by inserting a reed or cane into the trachea of animals.[16] In 1908 George Poe demonstrated his mechanical respirator by asphyxiating dogs and seemingly bringing them back to life.[17]

2.13.14 References

[1] GN-13: Guidance on the Risk Classification of General Medical Devices, Revision 1.1. From Health Sciences Authority. May 2014

[2] Parker JC, Hernandez LA, Peevy KJ (1993). "Mechanisms of ventilator-induced lung injury". *Crit Care Med* **21** (1): 131–43. doi:10.1097/00003246-199301000-00024. PMID 8420720.

[3] "International consensus conferences in intensive care medicine: Ventilator-associated Lung Injury in ARDS. This official conference report was cosponsored by the American Thoracic Society, The European Society of Intensive Care Medicine, and The Societé de Réanimation de Langue Française, and was approved by the ATS Board of Directors, July 1999". *Am. J. Respir. Crit. Care Med.* **160** (6): 2118–24. December 1999. doi:10.1164/ajrccm.160.6.ats16060. PMID 10588637.

[4] Levine S, Nguyen T, Taylor N, Friscia ME, Budak MT, Rothenberg P, et al. (2008). "Rapid disuse atrophy of diaphragm fibers in mechanically ventilated humans". *N Engl J Med* **358** (13): 1327–35. doi:10.1056/NEJMoa070447. PMID 18367735.

[5] De Jonghe B, Sharshar T, Lefaucheur JP, Authier FJ, Durand-Zaleski I, Boussarsar M, et al. (2002). "Paresis acquired in the intensive care unit: a prospective multicenter study". *JAMA* **288** (22): 2859–67. doi:10.1001/jama.288.22.2859. PMID 12472328.

[6] Konrad F, Schreiber T, Brecht-Kraus D, Georgieff M (1994). "Mucociliary transport in ICU patients". *Chest* **105** (1): 237–41. doi:10.1378/chest.105.1.237. PMID 8275739.

[7] Hess DR (2011). "Approaches to conventional mechanical ventilation of the patient with acute respiratory distress syndrome". *Respir Care* **56** (10): 1555–72. doi:10.4187/respcare.01387. PMID 22008397.

[8] Hoesch, Robert; Eric Lin; Mark Young; Rebecca Gottesman; Laith Altaweel; Paul Nyquist; Robert Stevens (February 2012). "Acute lung injury in critical neurological illness". *Critical care medicine* **40** (2): 587–593. doi:10.1097/CCM.0b013e3182329617. PMID 21946655.

[9] O'Connor HH (2011). "Prolonged mechanical ventilation: are you a lumper or a splitter?". *Respir Care* **56** (11): 1859–60. doi:10.4187/respcare.01600. PMID 22035828.

[10] Esteban A, Anzueto A, Alía I, Gordo F, Apezteguía C, Pálizas F, et al. (2000). "How is mechanical ventilation employed in the intensive care unit? An international utilization review.". *Am J Respir Crit Care Med* **161** (5): 1450–8. doi:10.1164/ajrccm.161.5.9902018. PMID 10806138.

[11] Yang KL, Tobin MJ (May 1991). "A prospective study of indexes predicting the outcome of trials of weaning from mechanical ventilation". *N. Engl. J. Med.* **324** (21): 1445–50. doi:10.1056/NEJM199105233242101. PMID 2023603.

[12] Tobin MJ (2006). *Principles and Practice of Mechanical Ventilation* (2nd ed.). McGraw Hill.

[13] Cook T, Howes B (December 2011). "Supraglottic airway devices: recent advances". *Contin Educ Anaesth Crit Care* **11** (2): 56–61. doi:10.1093/bjaceaccp/mkq058.

[14] Carley SD, Gwinnutt C, Butler J, Sammy I, Driscoll P (March 2002). "Rapid sequence induction in the emergency department: a strategy for failure". *Emerg Med J* **19** (2): 109–13. doi:10.1136/emj.19.2.109. PMC 1725832. PMID 11904254.

[15] Colice, Gene L (2006). "Historical Perspective on the Development of Mechanical Ventilation". In Martin J Tobin. *Principles & Practice of Mechanical Ventilation* (2 ed.). New York: McGraw-Hill. ISBN 978-0-07-144767-6.

[16] Chamberlain D (2003). "Never quite there: a tale of resuscitation medicine". *Clin Med* **3** (6): 573–7. doi:10.7861/clinmedicine.3-6-573. PMID 14703040.

[17] "Smother Small Dog To See it Revived. Successful Demonstration of an Artificial Respiration Machine Cheered in Brooklyn. Women in the Audience, But Most of Those Present Were Physicians. The Dog, Gathered in from the Street, Wagged Its Tail.". New York Times. May 29, 1908. Retrieved 2007-12-25. An audience, composed of about thirty men and three or four women, most of the men being physicians, attended a demonstration of Prof. George Poe's machine for producing artificial respiration in the library of the Kings County Medical Society, at 1,313 Bedford Avenue, Brooklyn, last night, under the auspices of the First Legion of the Red Cross Society.

2.13.15   External links

- e-Medicine, article on mechanical ventilation along with technical information.

- International Ventilator Users Network (IVUN), Resource of information for users of home mechanical ventilation.

2.14   Minimally conscious state

A **minimally conscious state** (**MCS**) is a disorder of consciousness distinct from persistent vegetative state and locked-in syndrome.   Unlike persistent vegetative state, patients with MCS have partial preservation of conscious awareness.[1] MCS is a relatively new category of disorders of consciousness. The natural history and longer term outcome of MCS have not yet been thoroughly studied. The prevalence of MCS was estimated to be 112,000 to 280,000 in adult and pediatric cases.[2]

2.14.1   History

Prior to the mid-1990s, there was a lack of operational definitions available to clinicians and researchers to guide the differential diagnosis among disorders of consciousness.   As a result, patients were lumped together into broad categories often based on the severity of the disability (e.g. moderate, severe, extremely severe). These diagnoses were performed without regard to salient differences in behavioral and pathological characteristics. In a three-year period spanning from 1994–1996, three position statements regarding the diagnostic criteria of disorder of consciousness were published. The "Medical Aspects of the Persistent Vegetative State" was published by the American Academy of Neurology (AAN) in 1994. In 1995, "Recommendations for Use of Uniform Nomenclature Pertinent to Patients With Severe Alterations in Consciousness" was published by the American Congress of Rehabilitation Medicine (ACRM). In 1996 the "International Working Party on the Management of the Vegetative State: Summary Report" was published by a group of international delegates from neurology, rehabilitation, neurosurgery, and neuropsychology. However, because the diagnostic criteria were published independently from one another, the final recommendations differed greatly from one another. The Aspen Neurobehavioral Work-group was convened to explore the underlying causes of these disparities. In the end, the Aspen Work-group provided a consensus statement regarding definitions and diagnostic criteria disorder of consciousness which include the vegetative state (VS) and the minimally conscious state (MCS).[3]

2.14.2   Definition and diagnostic criteria

Medical definition

Minimally conscious state (MCS) is defined as a condition of severely altered consciousness in which minimal but definite behavioral evidence of self or environmental awareness is demonstrated.[1]

Diagnosis

Although MCS patients are able to demonstrate cognitively mediated behavior, they occur inconsistently. They are, however, reproducible or can be sustained long enough to be differentiated from reflexive behavior. Because of this inconsistency, extended assessment may be required to determine if a simple response (e.g. a finger movement or a blink) occurred because of a specific environmental event (e.g. a command to move the finger or to blink) or was merely a coincidental behavior.[1] Distinguishing between VS and MCS is often difficult because the diagnosis is dependent on observation of behavior that show self or environmental awareness and because those behavioral responses are markedly reduced. One of the more common diagnostic errors involving disorders of consciousness is mistaking MCS for VS which may lead to serious repercussions related to clinical management.[4]

Giacino et al. have suggested demonstration of the following behaviors in order to make the diagnosis of MCS.

- Following simple commands.

- Gestural or verbal yes/no responses (regardless of accuracy).

- Intelligible verbalization.

- Purposeful behavior such as those that are contingent due to appropriate environmental stimuli and are not reflexive. Some examples of purposeful behavior include:

  - appropriate smiling or crying in response to the linguistic or visual content of emotional but not to neutral topics or stimuli.

  - vocalizations or gestures that occur in direct response to the linguistic content of questions.

  - reaching for objects that demonstrates a clear relationship between object location and direction of reach.

  - touching or holding objects in a manner that accommodates the size and shape of the object.

  - pursuit eye movement or sustained fixation that occurs in direct response to moving or salient stimuli.[1]

2.14.3 Prognosis

One of the defining characteristics of minimally conscious state is the more continuous improvement and significantly more favorable outcomes post injury when compared with vegetative state. One study looked at 100 patients with severe brain injury. At the beginning of the study, all the patients were unable to follow commands consistently or communicate reliably. These patients were diagnosed with either MCS or vegetative state based on performance on the JFK Coma Recovery Scale and the diagnostic criteria for MCS as recommended by the Aspen Consensus Conference Work-group. Both patient groups were further separated into those that suffered from traumatic brain injury and those that suffered from non-traumatic brain injures (anoxia, tumor, hydrocephalus, infection). The patients were assessed multiple times over a period of 12 months post injury using the Disability Rating Scale (DRS) which ranges from a score of 30=dead to 0=no disabilities. The results show that the DRS scores for the MCS subgroups showed the most improvement and predicted the most favorable outcomes 12 months post injury. Amongst those diagnosed with MCS, DRS scores were significantly lower for those with non-traumatic brain injuries in comparison to the vegetative state patients with traumatic brain injury. DRS scores were also significantly lower for the MCS non-traumatic brain injury group compared to the vegetative state non-traumatic brain injury group. Pairwise comparisons showed that DRS scores were significantly higher for those that suffered from non-tramuatic brain injuries than those with traumatic brain injuries. For the patients in vegetative states there were no significant differences between patients with non-traumatic brain injury and those with traumatic brain injuries. Out of the 100 patients studied, 3 patients fully recovered (had a DRS score of 0). These 3 patients were diagnosed with MCS and had suffered from traumatic brain injuries.[4]

In summary, those with minimally conscious state and non-traumatic brain injuries will not progress as well as those with traumatic brain injuries while those in vegetative states have an all around lower to minimal chance of recovery.

Because of the major differences in prognosis described in this study, this makes it crucial that MCS be diagnosed correctly. Incorrectly diagnosing MCS as vegetative state may lead to serious repercussions related to clinical management.

2.14.4 Pathophysiology

Neuroimaging

Because minimally conscious state has been a relatively new criteria for diagnosis, there are very few functional imaging studies of patients with this condition. Preliminary data has shown that overall cerebral metabolism is less than in those with conscious awareness (20-40% of normal[5]) and is slightly higher but comparable to those in vegetative states.

Activation in the medial parietal cortex and adjacent posterior cingulate cortex are brain regions that seem to differ between patients in MCS and those from vegetative states. These areas are most active during periods of conscious waking and are least active when in altered states of consciousness, such as general anesthesia, propofol, hypnotic state, dementia, and Wernicke–Korsakoff syndrome. Auditory stimulation induced more widespread activation in the primary and pre-frontal associative areas of MCS patients than vegetative state patients. There were also more cortio-cortical functional connectivity between the auditory cortex and a large network of temporal and prefrontal cortices in MCS than vegetative states. These findings encourage treatments based on neuromodulatory and cognitive revalidation therapeutic strategies for patients with MCS.[6]

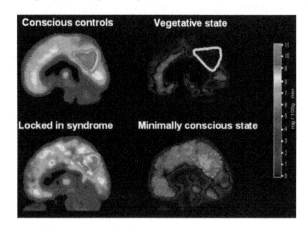

Resting overall cerebral metabolism of various brain states.[6]

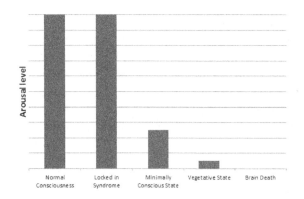

Arousal levels of various brain states.[6]

One study used diffusion tensor imaging (DTI) in two case studies. They found that there were widespread cerebral atrophy in both patients. The lateral ventricles were increased in size, and the corpus callosum and the periventricular white matter were diminished. The DTI maps showed that there was significant reduction of volume in the medial corpus callosum and other parts of the brain compared to normal subjects. They also found markedly lower diffusion

values in white matter and increased cerebral spinal fluid compartments. Cortical injuries at this level provides a particular favorable environment for sprouting of new axons to occur in the intact areas of the cortex, which may explain some of the greater recovery rates in minimally conscious state patients. The axonal regrowth has been correlated with functional motor recovery. The regrowth and rerouting of the axons may explain some of the changes to brain structure. These findings support the efforts to prospectively and longitudinally characterize neuroplasticity in both brain structure and function following severe injuries. Utilizing DTI and other neuroimaging techniques may further shed light on the debates on long-distance cortical rewiring and may lead to better rehabilitation strategies.[7]

Some areas of the brain that are correlated with the subjective experience of pain were activated in MCS patients when noxious stimulation was present. Positron emission tomography (PET) scans found increased blood flow to the secondary sensory cortex, posterior parietal cortex, premotor cortex, and the superior temporal cortex. The pattern of activation, however, was with less spatial extent. Some parts of the brain were less activated than normal patients during noxious stimulus processing. These were the posterior cingulate, medial prefrontal cortex, and the occipital cortex. Even though functional brain imaging can objectively measure changes in brain function during noxious stimulation, the role of different areas of the brain in pain processing is only partially understood. Furthermore, there is still the problem of the subjective experience. MCS patients by definition cannot consistently and reliably communicate their experiences. Even if they were able to answer the question "are you in pain?", there would not be a reliable response. Further clinical trials are needed to access the appropriateness of the use of analgesia in patients with MCS.[8]

Residual language function

A functional magnetic resonance imaging (fMRI) study found that minimally conscious state patients showed activation in auditory networks when they heard narratives that had personally meaningful content that were read forwards by a familiar voice. These activations were not seen when the narratives were read backwards.[9]

Another study compared patients in vegetative state and minimally conscious state in their ability to recognize language. They found that some patients in minimally conscious state demonstrated some evidence of preserved speech processing. There was more activation in response to sentences compared to white noise.[10]

2.14.5   Treatment

There is currently no definitive evidence that support altering the course of the recovery of minimally conscious state. There are currently multiple clinical trials underway investigating potential treatments.[11] In one case study, stimulation of thalamus using deep brain stimulation (DBS) lead to some behavioral improvements. The patient was a 38-year-old male who had remained in minimally conscious state following a severe traumatic brain injury. He had been unresponsive to consistent command following or communication ability and had remained non-verbal over two years in inpatient rehabilitation. fMRI scans showed preservation of a large-scale, bi-hemispheric cerebral language network, which indicates that possibility for further recovery may exist. Positron emission tomography showed that the patient's global cerebral metabolism levels were markedly reduced. He had DBS electrodes implanted bilaterally within his central thalamus.   More specifically, the DBS electrodes targeted the anterior intralaminar nuclei of thalamus and adjacent paralaminar regions of thalamic association nuclei.   Both electrodes were positioned within the central lateral nucleus, the paralaminar regions of the median dorsalis, and the posterior-medial aspect of the centromedian/parafasicularis nucleus complex. This allowed maximum coverage of the thalamic bodies. A DBS stimulation was conducted such that the patient was exposed to various patterns of stimulation to help identify optimal behavioral responses. Approximately 140 days after the stimulation began, qualitative changes in behavior emerged. There were longer periods of eye opening and increased responses to command stimuli as well as higher scores on the JFK coma recovery scale (CRS). Functional object use and intelligible verbalization was also observed. The observed improvements in arousal level, motor control, and consistency of behavior could be a result of direct activation of frontal cortical and basal ganglia systems that were innervated by neurons within the thalamic association nuclei. These neurons act as a key communication relay and form a pathway between the brainstem arousal systems and frontal lobe regions. This pathway is crucial for many executive functions such as working memory, effort regulation, selective attention, and focus.[12]

In another case study of a 50-year-old woman who had symptoms consistent with MCS, administration of zolpidem, a sedative hypnotic drug improved the patient's condition significantly.   Without treatment, the patient showed signs of mutism, athetoid movements of the extremities, and complete dependence for all personal care. 45 minutes after 5 to 10 mg of zolpidem was administered, the patient ceased the athetoid movements, regained speaking ability, and was able to self-feed. The effect lasted 3–4 hours from which she returned to the former state. The effects were repeated on a daily basis. PET scans showed that after zolpidem was administered, there was a marked increase in blood flow to areas of the brain adjacent to or distant from damaged tissues. In this case, these areas were the ipsilateral cerebral hemispheres and the cerebellum. These areas are thought to have been inhibited by the site of injury through a GABA-mediated mechanism and the inhibition was modified by zolpidem which is a GABA agonist. The fact that zolpidem is a sedative drug that induces sleep in normal people but causes arousal in a MCS patient is paradoxical. The mechanisms to why this effect occurs is not entirely clear.[13]

There is recent evidence that transcranial direct current stimulation (tDCS), a technique that supplies a small electric current in the brain with non-invasive electrodes, may improve the clinical state of patients with MCS. In one study with 10 patients with disorders of consciousness (7 in VS, 3 in MCS), tDCS was applied for 20 minutes every day for 10 days, and showed clinical improvement in all 3 patients who were in MCS, but not in those with VS. These results remained at 12-month follow-up. Two of the patients in MCS that had their brain insult less that 12 months recovered consciousness in the following months. One of these patients received a second round of tDCS treatment 4 months after his initial treatment, and showed further recovery and emerged into consciousness, with no change of clinical status between the two treatments.[14] Moreover, in a sham-controlled, double-blind crossover study, the immediate effects of a single session of tDCS were shown to transiently improve the clinical status of 13 out of 30 patients with MCS, but not in those with VS[15]

2.14.6   Ethical issues

One of the major ethical concerns involving patients with severe brain damage is their inability to communicate. By definition, patients who are unconscious or are minimally conscious are incapable of giving informed consent which is required for participation in clinical research. Typically, written approval is obtained from family members or legal representatives. The inability to receive informed consent has led to much research being refused grants, ethics committee approval, or research publication. This puts patients in these conditions at risk of being denied therapy that may be life-saving.[6]

The right to die

The right to die in patients with severe cognitive impairment has developed over time because of their grave neurological state and the perceived futility of continued treatment. Such cases have been debated vigorously in the past, as in the case with Terri Schiavo who was diagnosed with persistent vegetative state. In the case of minimally conscious state patients, they are neither permanently unconscious nor are they necessarily hopelessly damaged. Thus, these patients warrant additional evaluation.[16] On one hand, some argue that entertaining the possibility of intervention in some patients may erode the "right to die" moral obligation. Conversely, there is also fear that people may associate attitudes with higher-functioning people in minimally conscious state with people in persistent vegetative state, thus minimizing the value of their lives.[17]

Regulating therapeutic nihilism

Currently, risk aversion dominates the ethical landscape when research involves those with impaired decision-making abilities.[16] Fears of therapeutic adventurism has led to a disproportionate view about the under-appreciation of potential benefits and an overstatement of risks. Thus, recognizing this distortion is important in order to calculate the right balance between protecting vulnerable populations that cannot provide autonomous consent and potentially restorative clinical trials.[16]

2.14.7   Notable patients

- Terry Wallis[18]
- Chi Cheng
- Prince Friso of Orange-Nassau
- Michael Schumacher[19]

2.14.8   References

[1] Giacino JT, Ashwal S, Childs N, Cranford R, Jennett B, Katz DI, et al. (February 2002). "The minimally conscious state: definition and diagnostic criteria". *Neurology* **58** (3): 349–53. doi:10.1212/wnl.58.3.349. PMID 11839831.

[2] Strauss, DJ; Ashal S; Day SM; et al. (2000). "Life expectancy of children in vegetative and minimally conscious states". *Pediatric Neurol* **23**: 1–8.

[3] Giacino JT, Whyte J (2005). "The Vegetative and Minimally Conscious States". *J Head Trauma Rehabil* **20** (1): 30–50. doi:10.1097/00001199-200501000-00005. PMID 15668569.

[4] Giacino, JT; Kalmar K (1997). "The Vegetative and Minimally Conscious States: A comparison of Clinical Features and Functional Outcome". *J Head Trauma Rehabil* **12** (4): 36–51. doi:10.1097/00001199-199708000-00005.

[5] Schiff, ND; Rodriguez-Moreno D; Kamal A; Kim K; Giacino JT; Plum F; et al. (2005). "fMRI reveals large-scale network activation in minimally conscious patients". *Neurology* **64** (3): 514–523. doi:10.1212/01.WNL.0000150883.10285.44. PMID 15699384.

[6] Laureys S, Owen AM, Schiff ND (2004). "Brain function in coma, vegetative state, and related disorders". *The Lancet Neurology* **3** (9): 537–546. doi:10.1016/S1474-4422(04)00852-X.

[7] Voss, H. U.; Uluç, A. M.; Dyke, J. P.; Watts, R.; Kobylarz, E. J.; McCandliss, B. D.; Heier, L. A.; Beattie, B. J.; Hamacher, K. A.; Vallabhajosula, S.; Goldsmith, S. J.; Ballon, D.; Giacino, J. T.; Schiff, N. D. (2006). "Possible axonal regrowth in late recovery from the minimally conscious state". *Journal of Clinical Investigation* **116** (7): 2005–2011. doi:10.1172/JCI27021. PMC 1483160. PMID 16823492.

[8] Boly, M. L.; Faymonville, M. E.; Schnakers, C.; Peigneux, P.; Lambermont, B.; Phillips, C.; Lancellotti, P.; Luxen, A.; Lamy, M.; Moonen, G.; Maquet, P.; Laureys, S. (2008). "Perception of pain in the minimally conscious state with PET activation: An observational study". *The Lancet Neurology* **7** (11): 1013. doi:10.1016/S1474-4422(08)70219-9.

[9] Schiff, ND; Plum F; Rezai AR (2002). "Developing prosthetics to treat cognitive disabilities resulting from acquired brain injuries". *Neurol Res* **24**: 166–24.

[10] Coleman, MR; et al. (2007). "Do vegetative patients retain aspects of language? Evidence from fMRI". *Brain* **130** (Pt 10): 2494–2507. doi:10.1093/brain/awm170. PMID 17827174.

[11] NIH. "Clinicaltrials.gov".

[12] Laureys S, Owen AM, Schiff ND (August 2007). "Behavioural improvements with thalamic stimulation after severe traumatic brain injury". *Nature* **448** (7153): 600–603. doi:10.1038/nature06041. PMID 17671503.

[13] Shames, J. L.; Ring, H. (2008). "Transient Reversal of Anoxic Brain Injury–Related Minimally Conscious State After Zolpidem Administration: A Case Report". *Archives of Physical Medicine and Rehabilitation* **89** (2): 386–388. doi:10.1016/j.apmr.2007.08.137. PMID 18226667.

[14] Angelakis E, Liouta E, Andreadis N, Korfias S, Ktonas P, Stranjalis G, Sakas DE. (2014). Transcranial direct current stimulation (tDCS) effects in disorders of consciousness. Arch Phys Med Rehabil;95:283-9.

[15] Thibaut A, Bruno MA, Ledoux D, Demertzi A, Laureys S. tDCS in patients with disorders of consciousness: sham-controlled randomized double-blind study. *Neurology.* 2014;82(13):1112-8.

[16] Fins JJ (April 2003). "Constructing an ethical stereotaxy for severe brain injury: balancing risks, benefits and access". *Nature Reviews Neuroscience* **4** (4): 323–327. doi:10.1038/nrn1079.

[17] Coleman, D (2002). "The minimally conscious state: definition and diagnostic criteria". *Neurology* **58**: 506–507. doi:10.1212/wnl.58.3.506.

[18] CBSNews. "Awakenings: Return To Life". Retrieved 21 November 2011.

[19] Hall, Allan (2014-09-17). "Michael Schumacher receiving £100,000-a-week treatment from 15 specialists in Switzerland". *Daily Express*.

2.15 Organ donation

"Organ donor" redirects here. For the song by DJ Shadow, see Endtroducing......

Organ donation is the donation of biological tissue or an organ of the human body from a living or dead person to a living recipient in need of a transplantation. Transplantable organs and tissues are removed in a surgical procedure following a determination, based on the donor's medical and social history, of which are suitable for transplantation. Such procedures are termed allotransplantations, distinguish them from xenotransplantation, the transfer of animal organs into human bodies. As of June 21, 2013, there are 118,617 people waiting for life-saving organ transplants in the U.S. Of these, 96,645 await kidney transplants. While views of organ donation are positive there is a large gap between the numbers of registered donors compared to those awaiting organ donations on a global level.

In 2015, a baby with anencephaly who lived for only 100 minutes has donated his kidneys as the youngest organ donor to an adult with renal failure.[1] Within the same year, researchers from the Ganogen Research Institute transplanted human fetal kidneys from therapeutic abortions, including from fetuses with anencephaly, into animals for future transplantation into human patients.[2] The animals were able to survive on the human kidney alone, demonstrating both function and growth of the human organ. [3]

2.15.1 Legislation and global perspectives

The laws of different countries allow potential donors to permit or refuse donation, or give this choice to relatives. The frequency of donations varies among countries.

Opt-in versus opt-out

See also: Mandated choice

There are two main methods for determining voluntary consent: "opt in" (only those who have given explicit consent are donors) and "opt out" (anyone who has not refused is a donor). Opt-out legislative systems dramatically increase effective rates of consent for donation (the so-called default effect).[4] For example, Germany, which uses an opt-in system, has an organ donation consent rate of 12% among its population, while Austria, a country with a very similar culture and economic development, but which uses an opt-out system, has a consent rate of 99.98%.[4][5]

However, because of public policies, cultural, infrastructural and other factors, this does not always translate directly into increased effective rates of donation. In terms of effective organ donations, in some systems like Australia (14.9 donors per million, 337 donors in 2011), family members are required to give consent or refusal, or may veto a potential recovery even if the donor has consented.[6] Some countries with an opt-out system like Spain (36 effective donors per million inhabitants[7]) or Austria (21 donors/million) have high donor rates and some countries with opt-in systems like Germany (16 donors/million) or Greece (6 donors/million) have lower effective donation rates. The president of the Spanish National Transplant Organisation has acknowledged Spain's legislative approach is likely not the primary reason for the country's success in increasing the donor rates, starting in the 1990s.[8]

Consent process

One way organizations are attempting to gain more donors is looking at the consent process. There are two types of consent being looked at. Explicit consent consists of the donor giving direct consent through proper registration depending on the country.[9] The second consent process is presumed consent, which does not need direct consent from the donor or the next of kin.[9] Presumed consent assumes that donation would have been permitted by the potential donor if permission was pursued.[9] Of possible donors an estimated twenty five percent of families refuse to donate a loved one's organs.[10]

United States

Over 120,000 people in need of an organ are on the U.S. government waiting list.[11] This crisis within the United States is growing rapidly because on average there are only 30,000 transplants performed each year. More than 6,000 people die each year from lack of a donor organ, an average of 19 people a day. Between the years 1988 and 2006 the number of transplants doubled, but the number of patients waiting for an organ grew six times as large.[12] It has been estimated that the number of organs donated would double if every person with suitable organs decided to donate. In the past presumed consent was urged to try to decrease the need for organs. The Uniform Anatomical Gift Act of 1987 was adopted in several states, and allowed medical examiners to determine if organs and tissues of cadavers could be donated. By the 1980s, several states adopted different laws that allowed only certain tissues or organs to be retrieved and donated, some allowed all, and some did not allow any without consent of the family. In 2006 when the UAGA was revised, the idea of presumed consent was abandoned. In the United States today, organ donation is done only with consent of the family or donator themselves.[13] In some cases doctors are reportedly removing pieces of tissue from already dead patients without consulting the patient of their families' consent. This is completely legal procedure. According to economist, Alex Tabarrok the shortage of organs has increased the use of so-called expanded criteria organs, or organs that used to be considered unsuitable for transplant.[14] Due to the lack of donation it is leading some countries to try unconventional practice, creating a lot of controversy and loss of money. The University of Maryland's School of Medicine there were five patients that received kidney transplants that obtained cancerous or benign tumors that were withdrawn from the organ. This raised many questions for the head surgeon, Dr. Michael Phelan who explained that "the ongoing shortage of organs from deceased donors, and the high risk of dying while waiting for a transplant, prompted five donors and recipients to push ahead with the surgery."[14] Doctors are becoming desperate and are having to use organs from patients who are over the age of 60. These donors have had multiple medical problems and are more likely to fail than those of a younger healthier donor.The certainty remains true that are more than 100,000 people waiting for a transplant. The number of recipients is growing faster than there are donors.

Argument for opt-out organ donation in the United States   Many Americans believe that what happens to their bodies after death should be solely up to them and for a long time this is how it has been. However, this is actually a very common misconception. The U.S. government already conducts autopsies after ambiguous deaths in which they remove large pieces of the person's internal organs for analysis and criminal investigation. Some would argue that if procedures such as this one are already being done then why not change the system all-together; even if it means dramatically changing current and deep rooted beliefs about the sanctity of human bodies. Changing the United States from an opt-in to an opt-out system would be an effective solution to the imbalance of those who are in need of organs and the amount of donors. For every 90,000 people who need kidneys there are only about 14,000 peo-

ple who are willing to donate. If the United States became an opt-out country its availability of organs could raise by up to 50%. There is already a push for a change in policy being made by several organizations such as the American Kidney Fund.[15]

Financial reward   In 1994 a bill was signed into law in Pennsylvania which proposed an idea that would increase the supply of organs for everyone. They decided to start paying $300 towards room and board and $3,000 to go towards funeral expenses to a donor's family. Officials went back and forth for eight years before deciding on this program. It is the first of its kind. Procurement directors and surgeons across the nation are now looking at Pennsylvania's program and watching for success.[16] Some are already planning to follow in its footsteps if this new incentive proves itself. There has already been at least nineteen families that have signed up for the benefit and there are more expected to come. There are people out there who oppose this plan fundamentally. One argument is it will disproportionately affect the poor.[17] The $300–3,000 reward will act as more incentive to the poor as opposed to the rich who may not find that amount of money to be worth it. Others may say that this new law in Pennsylvania violates the integrity of the self.

Europe

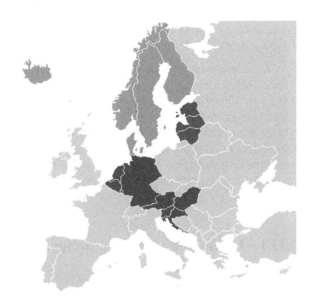

Map showing the coverage of 3 international European organ donation associations: Balttransplant, Eurotransplant and Scandiatransplant

Within the European Union, organ donation is regulated by member states. As of 2010, 24 European countries have some form of presumed consent (opt-out) system, with the most prominent and limited opt-out systems in Spain, Austria, and Belgium yielding high donor rates.[18] In the United Kingdom organ donation is voluntary and no consent is presumed. Individuals who wish to donate their organs after death can use the Organ Donation Register, a national database. The government of Wales became the first constituent country in the UK to adopt presumed consent in July 2013.[19] In 2008, the UK discussed whether to switch to an opt-out system in light of the success in other countries and a severe British organ donor shortfall.[20] In Italy if the deceased neither allowed nor refused donation while alive, relatives will pick the decision on his or her behalf despite a 1999 act that provided for a proper opt-out system.[21] In 2008, the European Parliament overwhelmingly voted for an initiative to introduce an EU organ donor card in order to foster organ donation in Europe.

Landstuhl Regional Medical Center (LRMC) has become one of the most active organ donor hospitals in all of Germany, which otherwise has one of the lowest organ donation participation rates in the Eurotransplant organ network. LRMC, the largest U.S. military hospital outside the United States, is one of the top hospitals for organ donation in the Rhineland-Palatinate state of Germany, even though it has relatively few beds compared to many German hospitals. According to the German organ transplantation organization, Deutsche Stiftung Organtransplantation (DSO), 34 American military service members who died at LRMC (roughly half of the total number who died there) donated a total of 142 organs between 2005 and 2010. In 2010 alone, 10 of the 12 American service members who died at LRMC were donors, donating a total of 45 organs. Of the 205 hospitals in the DSO's central region—which includes the large cities of Frankfurt and Mainz—only six had more organ donors than LRMC in 2010.[22]

Japan

See also: Organ transplantation in Japan

The rate of organ donation in Japan is significantly lower than in Western countries.[23] This is attributed to cultural reasons, some distrust of western medicine, and a controversial organ transplantation in 1968 that provoked a ban on cadaveric organ donation that would last thirty years.[23] Organ donation in Japan is regulated by a 1997 organ transplant law, which defines "brain death" and legalized organ procurement from brain dead donors.

India

India has a fairly well developed corneal donation programme however donation after brain death has been rel-

atively slow to take off. Most of the transplants done in India are living related or unrelated transplants. To curb organ commerce and promote donation after brain death the government enacted a law called "The Transplantation of Human Organs Act" in 1994 that brought about a significant change in the organ donation and transplantation scene in India. [24][25][26][27] [28][29][30][31][32] Many Indian states have adopted the law and in 2011 further amendment of the law took place.[33][34][35][36] [37] Despite the law there have been stray instances of organ trade in India and these have been widely reported in the press. This resulted in the amendment of the law further in 2011. Deceased donation after brain death have slowly started happening in India and 2012 was the best year for the programme.

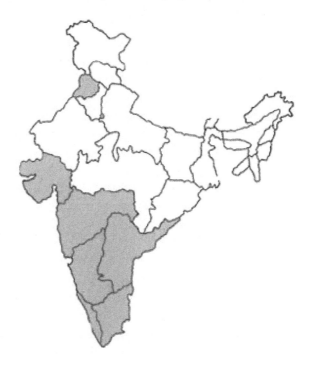

Map shows Indian states that have done Deceased Donation Transplantation in India

Source: Indian Transplant News Letter of MOHAN Foundation (Vol 2 Issue No. 37 of 2013)

The year 2013 has been the best yet for deceased organ donation in India. A total of 845 organs were retrieved from 310 multi-organ donors resulting in a national organ donation rate of 0.26 per million population(Table 2).

* ODR (pmp) – Organ Donation Rate (per million population)

In the year 2000 through the efforts of an NGO called MOHAN Foundation state of Tamil Nadu started an organ sharing network between a few hospitals.[38][39] This NGO also set up similar sharing network in the state of Andhra Pradesh and these two states were at the forefront of deceased donation and transplantation programme for many years.[40][41] As a result, retrieval of 1033 organs and tissues were facilitated in these two states by the NGO.[42] Similar sharing networks came up in the states of Maharastra and Karnataka; however the numbers of deceased donation happening in these states were not sufficient to make much impact.

In 2008, the Government of Tamil Nadu put together government orders laying down procedures and guidelines for deceased organ donation and transplantation in the state.[43] These brought in almost thirty hospitals in the programme and has resulted in significant increase in the donation rate in the state. With an organ donation rate of 1.15 per million population, Tamil Nadu is the leader in deceased organ donation in the country. The small success of Tamil Nadu model has been possible due to the coming together of both government and private hospitals, NGOs and the State Health department. Most of the deceased donation programmes have been developed in southern states of India.[44]

The various such programmes are as follows-

- Andhra Pradesh - Jeevandan programme

- Karnataka - Zonal Coordination Committee of Karnataka for Transplantation

- Kerala - Mrithasanjeevani - The Kerala Network for Organ Sharing

- Maharashtra - Zonal Transplant Coordination Center in Mumbai

- Tamil Nadu – Cadaver Transplant Programme

In the year 2012 besides Tamil Nadu other southern states too did deceased donation transplants more frequently. An online organ sharing registry for deceased donation and transplantation is used by the states of Tamil Nadu (www.tnos.org) and Kerala (www.knos.org.in). Both these registries have been developed, implemented and maintained by MOHAN Foundation.

Organ selling is legally banned in Asia. Numerous studies have documented that organ vendors have a poor *quality of life* (QOL) following kidney donation. However a study done by Vemuru reddy *et al* shows a significant improvement in Quality of life contrary to the earlier belief.[45] Live related renal donors have a significant improvement in the QOL following renal donation using the WHO QOL BREF in a study done at the All India Institute of Medical Sciences from 2006 to 2008. The quality of life of the donor was poor when the graft was lost or the recipient died.[45]

Sri Lanka

Organ donation in Sri Lanka was ratified by the Human Tissue Transplantation Act No. 48 of 1987. Sri Lanka Eye Donation Society, a non-governmental organization established in 1961 has provided over 60,000 corneas for corneal transplantation, for patients in 57 countries. It is one of the major suppliers of human eyes to the world, with a supply of approximately 3,000 corneas per year.[46]

Israel

See also: Organ transplantation in Israel

Since 2008, signing an organ donor card in Israel has provided a potential medical benefit to the signer. If two patients require an organ donation and have the same medical need, preference will be given to the one that had signed an organ donation card. This policy was nicknamed "dont give, don't get". Organ donation in Israel increased after 2008.

Brazil

A campaign by Sport Club Recife has led to waiting lists for organs in north-east Brazil to drop almost to zero; while according to the Brazilian law the family has the ultimate authority, the issuance of the organ donation card and the ensuing discussions have however eased the process.[47]

New Zealand

New Zealand law allows live donors to participate in altruistic organ donation only. In 2013 there were 3 cases of liver donation by live donors and 58 cases of kidney donation by live donors.[48] New Zealand has low rates of live donation, which could be due to the fact that it is illegal to pay someone for their organs. The Human Tissue Act 2008 states that trading in human tissue is prohibited, and is punishable by a fine of up to $50,000 or a prison term of up to 1 year.[49]

New Zealand law also allows for organ donation from deceased individuals. In 2013 organs were taken from 36 deceased individuals.[50] Everyone who applies for a drivers license in New Zealand indicates whether or not they wish to be a donor if they die in circumstances that would allow for donation.[51] The question is required to be answered for the application to be processed, meaning that the individual must answer yes or no, and does not have the option of leaving it unanswered.[51] However, the answer given on the drivers license does not constitute informed consent, because at the time of drivers license application not all individuals are equipped to make an informed decision regarding whether to be a donor, and it is therefore not the deciding factor in whether donation is carried out or not.[51] It is there to simply give indication of the person's wishes.[51] Family must agree to the procedure for donation to take place.[51][52]

A 2006 bill proposed setting up an organ donation register where people can give informed consent to organ donations and clearly state their legally binding wishes.[53] However, the bill did not pass, and there was condemnation of the bill from some doctors, who said that even if a person had given express consent for organ donation to take place, they would not carry out the procedure in the presence of any disagreement from grieving family members.[54]

The indigenous population of New Zealand also have strong views regarding organ donation. Many Maori people believe organ donation is morally unacceptable due to the cultural need for a dead body to remain fully intact.[55] However, because there is not a universally recognised cultural authority, no one view on organ donation is universally accepted in the Maori population.[55] They are, however, less likely to accept a kidney transplant than other New Zealanders, despite being overrepresented in the population receiving dialysis.[55]

2.15.2 Iran

Only one country, Iran has eliminated the shortage of transplant organs - and only Iran has a working and legal payment system for organ donation. [54] It is also the only country where organ trade is legal. The way their system works is, if a patient does not have a living relative or who are not assigned an organ from a deceased donor, apply to the nonprofit Dialysis and Transplant Patients Association (Datpa). The association establishes potential donors, those donors are assessed by transplant doctors who are not affiliated with the Datpa association. The government gives a compensation of $1,200 to the donors and aid them a year of limited health-insurance. Additionally, working through Datpa, kidney recipients pay donors between $2,300 and $4,500.[14] Importantly, it is illegal for the medical and surgical teams involved or any 'middleman' to receive payment.[56] Charity donations are made to those donors whose recipients are unable to pay. The Iranian system began in 1988 and eliminated the shortage of kidneys by 1999. Within the first year of the establishment of this system, the number of transplants had almost doubled; nearly four fifths were from living unrelated sources.[56][55] This system has exhibited a way to stop organ shortage. Which is to reimburse living donors for their organs. Other countries need to observe this method in the

hopes that they will be able to alleviate the lack of organ donors. Nobel Laureate economist Gary Becker and Julio Elias estimated that a payment of $15,000 for living donors would alleviate the shortage of kidneys in the U.S.[14]

2.15.3 Bioethical issues

Deontological issues

Certain groups, like the Roma (gypsies), oppose organ donation on religious grounds, but most of the world's religions support donation as a charitable act of great benefit to the community.[57] Issues surrounding patient autonomy, living wills, and guardianship make it nearly impossible for involuntary organ donation to occur.

From the standpoint of deontological ethics, the primary issues surrounding the morality of organ donation are semantical in nature. The debate over the definitions of life, death, human, and body is ongoing. For example, whether or not a brain-dead patient ought to be kept artificially animate in order to preserve organs for procurement is an ongoing problem in clinical bioethics. In addition, some have argued that organ donation constitutes an act of self-harm, even when an organ is donated willingly.

Further, the use of cloning to produce organs with an identical genotype to the recipient has issues all its own. Cloning is still a controversial topic, especially considering the possibility for an entire person to be brought into being with the express purpose of being destroyed for organ procurement. While the benefit of such a cloned organ would be a zero-percent chance of transplant rejection, the ethical issues involved with creating and killing a clone may outweigh these benefits. However, it may be possible in the future to use cloned stem-cells to grow a new organ without creating a new human being.

A relatively new field of transplantation has reinvigorated the debate. Xenotransplantation, or the transfer of animal (usually pig) organs into human bodies, promises to eliminate many of the ethical issues, while creating many of its own. While xenotransplantation promises to increase the supply of organs considerably, the threat of organ transplant rejection and the risk of xenozoonosis, coupled with general anathema to the idea, decreases the functionality of the technique. Some animal rights groups oppose the sacrifice of an animal for organ donation and have launched campaigns to ban them.

Teleological issues

On teleological or utilitarian grounds, the moral status of "black market organ donation" relies upon the ends, rather than the means. In so far as those who donate organs are often impoverished and those who can afford black market organs are typically well-off, it would appear that there is an imbalance in the trade. In many cases, those in need of organs are put on waiting lists for *legal* organs for indeterminate lengths of time — many die while still on a waiting list.

Organ donation is fast becoming an important bioethical issue from a social perspective as well. While most first-world nations have a legal system of oversight for organ transplantation, the fact remains that demand far outstrips supply. Consequently, there has arisen a black market trend often referred to as *transplant tourism.* The issues are weighty and controversial. On the one hand are those who contend that those who can afford to buy organs are exploiting those who are desperate enough to sell their organs. Many suggest this results in a growing inequality of status between the rich and the poor. On the other hand are those who contend that the desperate should be allowed to sell their organs and that preventing them from doing so is merely contributing to their status as impoverished. Further, those in favor of the trade hold that exploitation is morally preferable to death, and in so far as the choice lies between abstract notions of justice on the one hand and a dying person whose life could be saved on the other hand, the organ trade should be legalized. Conversely, surveys conducted among living donors postoperatively and in a period of five years following the procedure have shown extreme regret in a majority of the donors, who said that given the chance to repeat the procedure, they would not.[58] Additionally, many study participants reported a decided worsening of economic condition following the procedure.[59] These studies looked only at people who sold a kidney in countries where organ sales are already legal.

A consequence of the black market for organs has been a number of cases and suspected cases of organ theft,[60][61] including murder for the purposes of organ theft.[62][63] Proponents of a legal market for organs say that the black-market nature of the current trade allows such tragedies and that regulation of the market could prevent them. Opponents say that such a market would encourage criminals by making it easier for them to claim that their stolen organs were legal.

Legalization of the organ trade carries with it its own sense of justice as well. Continuing black-market trade creates further disparity on the demand side: only the rich can afford such organs. Legalization of the international organ trade could lead to increased supply, lowering prices so that persons outside the wealthiest segments could afford such organs as well.

Exploitation arguments generally come from two main areas:

- *Physical exploitation* suggests that the operations in question are quite risky, and, taking place in third-world hospitals or "back-alleys," even more risky. Yet, if the operations in question can be made safe, there is little threat to the donor.

- *Financial exploitation* suggests that the donor (especially in the Indian subcontinent and Africa) are not paid enough. Commonly, accounts from persons who have sold organs in both legal and black market circumstances put the prices at between $150 and $5,000, depending on the local laws, supply of ready donors and scope of the transplant operation.[64][65][66] In Chennai, India where one of the largest black markets for organs is known to exist, studies have placed the average sale price at little over $1,000.[59] Many accounts also exist of donors being postoperatively denied their promised pay.[67]

The New Cannibalism is a phrase coined by anthropologist Nancy Scheper-Hughes in 1998 for an article written for The New Internationalist. Her argument was that the actual exploitation is an ethical failing, a human exploitation; a perception of the poor as organ sources which may be used to extend the lives of the wealthy.[68]

Economic drivers leading to increased donation are not limited to areas such as India and Africa, but also are emerging in the United States. Increasing funeral expenses combined with decreasing real value of investments such as homes and retirement savings which took place in the 2000s have purportedly led to an increase in citizens taking advantage of arrangements where funeral costs are reduced or eliminated.[69]

Brain death versus cardiac death

Brain death may result in legal death, but still with the heart beating, and with mechanical ventilation, all other vital organs may be kept alive and functional for a certain period of time. Given long enough, patients who do not fully die, in the complete biological sense, but who are declared brain dead will usually, either after a shorter or longer interval, depending upon the patient's case and the type and extent of trauma and their age and prior health, start to build up toxins and wastes in the body, and the organs (especially sensitive ones like the brain, nerves, heart, blood vessels, lungs, liver, intestines, and kidneys) eventually can dysfunction, have coagulopathies or fluid and electrolyte and nutrient imbalances, or even fail- partially, or completely and irreversibly. Thus, the organs will usually only be sustainable and viable for acceptable use up until a certain length of time (most organs that are transplanted fortunately have widely used and agreed upon parameters, that are measurable and reliable, when determining their welfare and level of function).

This will depend on how well the patient is maintained, any other comorbidities, the skill of the medical, nursing, and surgical teams, and the quality of the care and the facilities- and once removed, the time and the mode of transport and how smoothly the transplant procedure (and the care before, during, and after the operation[s]), goes.[70] Given optimal care and oversight, and with the person's (through a directive or driver's license) and/or guardian or next of kin or power of attorney's informed consent, certain cases can provide optimal opportunities for organ transplantation. A major point of contention is whether transplantation should be allowed at all if the patient is not yet fully (biologically) dead, and if brain death is acceptable, whether the person's whole brain needs to have died, or if the death of a part of the brain (i.e., the cerebrum- which makes us human in our intellectual, and indeed all, conscious capacities; or the brain stem- which controls vital organic functions needed for life, like breathing and precise heartbeat regulation) is enough for legal and ethical and moral purposes.

Most organ donation for organ transplantation is done in the setting of brain death. However, in Japan this is a fraught point, and prospective donors may designate either brain death or cardiac death – see organ transplantation in Japan. In some nations (for instance, Belgium, Poland, Portugal and France) everyone is automatically an organ donor, although some jurisdictions (such as Singapore, Portugal, Poland,or New Zealand) allow opting out of the system. Elsewhere, consent from family members or next-of-kin is required for organ donation. The non-living donor is kept on ventilator support until the organs have been surgically removed. If a brain-dead individual is not an organ donor, ventilator and drug support is discontinued and cardiac death is allowed to occur.

In the United States, where since the 1980s the Uniform Determination of Death Act has defined death as the irreversible cessation of the function of either the brain or the heart and lungs,[71] the 21st century has seen an order-of-magnitude increase of donation following cardiac death. In 1995, only one out of 100 dead donors in the nation gave their organs following the declaration of cardiac death. That figure grew to almost 11 percent in 2008, according to the Scientific Registry of Transplant Recipients.[71] That increase has provoked ethical concerns about the interpretation of "irreversible" since "patients may still be alive five or even 10 minutes after cardiac arrest because, theoretically, their hearts could be restarted, [and thus are] clearly not dead because their condition was reversible."[71]

2.15.4 Political issues

There are also controversial issues regarding how organs are allocated to recipients. For example, some believe that livers should not be given to alcoholics in danger of reversion, while others view alcoholism as a medical condition like diabetes.

Faith in the medical system is important to the success of organ donation. Brazil switched to an opt-out system and ultimately had to withdraw it because it further alienated patients who already distrusted the country's medical system.[72]

Adequate funding, strong political will to see transplant outcomes improve, and the existence of specialized training, care and facilities also increase donation rates. Expansive legal definitions of death, such as Spain uses, also increase the pool of eligible donors by allowing physicians to declare a patient to be dead at an earlier stage, when the organs are still in good physical condition.

Allowing or forbidding payment for organs affects the availability of organs. Generally, where organs cannot be bought or sold, quality and safety are high, but supply is not adequate to the demand. Where organs can be purchased, the supply increases.[73]

> Iran adopted a system of paying kidney donors in 1988 and within 11 years it became the only country in the world to clear its waiting list for transplants.
> — The Economist

Healthy humans have two kidneys, a redundancy{{http://www.scientificamerican.com/article/how-can-you-live-without/ldate=August 2014}} that enables living donors (*inter vivos*) to give a kidney to someone who needs it. The most common transplants are to close relatives, but people have given kidneys to other friends. The rarest type of donation is the undirected donation whereby a donor gives a kidney to a stranger. Less than a few hundred of such kidney donations have been performed. In recent years, searching for altruistic donors via the internet has also become a way to find life saving organs. However, internet advertising for organs is a highly controversial practice, as some scholars believe it undermines the traditional list-based allocation system.[74]

The National Transplant Organization of Spain is one of the most successful in the world, but it still cannot meet the demand, as 10% of those needing a transplant die while still on the transplant list.[75] Donations from corpses are anonymous, and a network for communication and transport allows fast extraction and transplant across the country. Under Spanish law, every corpse can provide organs unless the deceased person had expressly rejected it. Because family members still can forbid the donation,[76] carefully trained doctors ask the family for permission, making it very similar in practice to the United States system.[77]

In the overwhelming majority of cases, organ donation is not possible for reasons of recipient safety, match failures, or organ condition. Even in Spain, which has the highest organ donation rate in the world, there are only 35.1 actual donors per million people, and there are hundreds of patients on the waiting list.[72] This rate compares to 24.8 per million in Austria, where families are rarely asked to donate organs, and 22.2 per million in France, which—like Spain—has a presumed-consent system.

Prison inmates

See also: Organ donation in the United States prison population

In the United States, prisoners are not discriminated against as organ recipients and are equally eligible for organ transplants along with the general population. A 1976 U.S. Supreme Court case[78] ruled that withholding health care from prisoners constituted "cruel and unusual punishment". United Network for Organ Sharing, the organization that coordinates available organs with recipients, does not factor a patient's prison status when determining suitability for a transplant.[79][80] An organ transplant and follow-up care can cost the prison system up to one million dollars.[80][81] If a prisoner qualifies, a state may allow compassionate early release to avoid high costs associated with organ transplants.[80] However, an organ transplant may save the prison system substantial costs associated with dialysis and other life-extending treatments required by the prisoner with the failing organ. For example, the estimated cost of a kidney transplant is about $111,000.[82] A prisoner's dialysis treatments are estimated to cost a prison $120,000 per year.[83]

Because donor organs are in short supply, there are more people waiting for a transplant than available organs. When a prisoner receives an organ, there is a high probability that someone else will die waiting for the next available organ. A response to this ethical dilemma states that felons who have a history of violent crime, who have violated others' basic rights, have lost the right to receive an organ transplant, though it is noted that it would be necessary "to reform our justice system to minimize the chance of an innocent person being wrongly convicted of a violent crime and thus being denied an organ transplant"[84]

Prisons typically do not allow inmates to donate organs to anyone but immediate family members. There is no law against prisoner organ donation; however, the transplant community has discouraged use of prisoner's organs since the early 1990s due to concern over prisons' high-risk environment for infectious diseases.[85] Physicians and ethicists also criticize the idea because a prisoner is not able to consent to the procedure in a free and non-coercive environment,[86] especially if given inducements to participate. However, with modern testing advances to more safely rule out infectious disease and by ensuring that there are no incentives offered to participate, some have argued that prisoners can now voluntarily consent to organ donation just as they can now consent to medical procedures in general. With careful safeguards, and with over 2 million prisoners in the U.S., they reason that prisoners can provide a solution for reducing organ shortages in the U.S.[87]

While some have argued that prisoner participation would likely be too low to make a difference, one Arizona program started by Maricopa County Sheriff Joe Arpaio encourages inmates to voluntarily sign up to donate their heart and other organs.[88] As of mid-2012, over 10,000 inmates had signed up in that one county alone.[89]

2.15.5 Religious viewpoints

Main article: Religious views on organ donation
See also: Organ donation in Jewish law

All major religions accept organ donation in at least some form on either utilitarian grounds (*i.e.*, because of its life-saving capabilities) or deontological grounds (*e.g.*, the right of an individual believer to make his or her own decision). Most religions, among them the Roman Catholic Church, support organ donation on the grounds that it constitutes an act of charity and provides a means of saving a life, consequently Pope Francis is an organ donor. One religious group, The Jesus Christians, became known as "The Kidney Cult" because more than half its members had donated their kidneys altruistically. Jesus Christians claim altruistic kidney donation is a great way to "Do unto others what they would want you to do unto them."[90] Some religions impose certain restrictions on the types of organs that may be donated and/or on the means by which organs may be harvested and/or transplanted.[91] For example, Jehovah's Witnesses require that organs be drained of any blood due to their interpretation of the Hebrew Bible/Christian Old Testament as prohibiting blood transfusion,[92] and Muslims require that the donor have provided written consent in advance.[92] A few groups disfavor organ transplantation or donation; notably, these include Shinto[93] and those who follow the customs of the Gypsies.[92]

Orthodox Judaism considers organ donation obligatory if it will save a life, as long as the donor is considered dead as defined by Jewish law.[92] In both Orthodox Judaism and non-Orthodox Judaism, the majority view holds that organ donation is permitted in the case of irreversible cardiac rhythm cessation. In some cases, rabbinic authorities believe that organ donation may be mandatory, whereas a minority opinion considers any donation of a live organ as forbidden.[94]

2.15.6 Organ shortfall

The demand for organs significantly surpasses the number of donors everywhere in the world. There are more potential recipients on organ donation waiting lists than organ donors. In particular, due to significant advances in dialysis techniques, patients suffering from end-stage renal disease (ESRD) can survive longer than ever before. Because these patients don't die as quickly as they used to, and as kidney failure increases with the rising age and prevalence of high blood pressure and diabetes in a society, the need especially for kidneys rises every year.

As of March 2014, about 121,600 people in the United States are on the waiting list, although about a third of those patients are inactive and could not receive a donated organ.[95][96] Wait times and success rates for organs differ significantly between organs due to demand and procedure difficulty. As of 2007, three-quarters of patients in need of an organ transplant were waiting for a kidney,[97] and as such kidneys have much longer waiting times. At the Oregon Health and Science University, for example, the median patient who ultimately received an organ waited only three weeks for a heart and three months for a pancreas or liver — but 15 months for a kidney, because demand for kidneys substantially outstrips supply.[98]

In Australia, there are 10.8 transplants per million people,[99] about a third of the Spanish rate. The Lions Eye Institute, in Western Australia, houses the Lions Eye Bank. The Bank was established in 1986 and coordinates the collection, processing and distribution of eye tissue for transplantation. The Lions Eye Bank also maintains a waitlist of patients who require corneal graft operations. About 100 corneas are provided by the Bank for transplant each year, but there is still a waiting list for corneas.[100]

"To an economist, this is a basic supply-and-demand gap with tragic consequences."[101] Approaches to addressing this shortfall include:

- donor registries and "primary consent" laws, to remove the burden of the donation decision from the legal next-of-kin. Illinois adopted a policy of "mandated choice" in 2006, which requires driver's license registrants to answer the question "Do you want to be an organ donor?" Illinois has a registration rate of 60 percent compared to 38 percent nationally.[102] The added cost of adding a question to the registration form is minimal.

- monetary incentives for signing up to be a donor.

Some economists have advocated going as far as allowing the sale of organs. The New York Times reported that "Gary Becker and Julio Jorge Elias argued in a recent paper that 'monetary incentives would increase the supply of organs for transplant sufficiently to eliminate the very large queues in organ markets, and the suffering and deaths of many of those waiting, without increasing the total cost of transplant surgery by more than 12 percent.'"[101] Iran allows the sale of kidneys, and has no waiting list.[103] The primary argument against this proposal is a moral one; as the article notes, many find such a suggestion repugnant.[101] As the National Kidney Foundation puts it, "Offering direct or indirect economic benefits in exchange for organ donation is inconsistent with our values as a society. Any attempt to assign a monetary value to the human body, or body parts, either arbitrarily, or through market forces, diminishes human dignity."[104]

- an opt-out system ("dissent solution"), in which a potential donor or his/her relatives must take specific action to be excluded from organ donation, rather than specific action to be included. This model is used in several European countries, such as Austria, which has a registration rate eight times that of Germany, which uses an opt-in system.[102]

- social incentive programs, wherein members sign a legal agreement to direct their organs first to other members who are on the transplant waiting list. One example of a private organization using this model is LifeSharers, which is free to join and whose members agree to sign a document giving preferred access to their organs.[105] "The proposal [for an organ mutual insurance pool] can be easily summarized: An individual would receive priority for any needed transplant if that individual agrees that his or her organs will be available to other members of the insurance pool in the event of his or her death. ... The main purpose [of this proposal] is to increase the supply of transplantable organs in order to save or improve more lives."[106]

In hospitals, organ network representatives routinely screen patient records to identify potential donors shortly in advance of their deaths.[107] In many cases, organ-procurement representatives will request screening tests (such as blood typing) or organ-preserving drugs (such as blood pressure drugs) to keep potential donors' organs viable until their suitability for transplants can be determined and family consent (if needed) can be obtained.[107] This practice increases transplant efficiency, as potential donors who are unsuitable due to infection or other causes are removed from consideration before their deaths, and decreases the avoidable loss of organs.[107] It may also benefit families indirectly, as the families of unsuitable donors are not approached to discuss organ donation.[107]

The Center for Ethical Solutions, an American bioethics think tank, is currently working on a project called "Solving the Organ Shortage," in which it is studying the Iranian kidney procurement system in order to better inform the debate over solving the organ shortfall in the United States.[108]

2.15.7   Distribution

The United States has two agencies that govern organ procurement and distribution within the country. The United Network for Organ Sharing and the Organ Procurement and Transplant Network (OPTN) regulate Organ Procurement Organizations (OPO) with regard to procurement and distribution ethics and standards. OPOs are non-profit organizations charged with the evaluation, procurement and allocation of organs whithin their Designated Service Area (DSA). Once a donor has been evaluated and consent obtained, provisional allocation of organs commences. UNOS developed a computer program that automatically generates donor specific match lists for suitable recipients based on the criteria that the patient was listed with. OPO coordinators enter donor information into the program and run the respective lists. Organ offers to potential recipients are made to transplant centers to make them aware of a potential organ. The surgeon will evaluate the donor information and make a provisional determination of medical suitability to their recipient. Distribution varies slightly between different organs but is essentially very similar. When lists are generated many factors are taken into consideration; these factors include: distance of transplant center from the donor hospital, blood type, medical urgency, wait time, donor size and tissue typing. For heart recipients medical urgency is denoted by a recipients "Status" (Status 1A, 1B and status 2). Lungs are allocated based on a recipients Lung Allocation Score (LAS) that is determined based on urgency and wait time. Livers are allocated using both a status system and MELD/PELD score (Model for End-stage Liver Disease/Pediatric End-stage Liver Disease). Kidney and pancreas lists are based on location, blood type, Human Leukocyte Antigen (HLA) typing and wait time. When a recipient for a kidney or pancreas has no direct antibodies to the donor HLA the match is said to be a 0 ABDR mismatch or zero antigen mismatch. A zero mismatch organ has a low rate of rejection and allows a recipient to be on lower doses of immunosuppressive drugs. Since zero mismatches have such high graft survival these recipients are afforded priority regardless of location and wait time. UNOS has in place a "Payback" system to balance organs that are sent out of a DSA because of a zero mismatch.

Location of a transplant center with respect to a donor hospital is given priority due to the effects of Cold Ischemic Time (CIT). Once the organ is removed from the donor, blood no longer perfuses through the vessels and begins to starve the cells of oxygen (ischemia). Each organ tolerates different ischemic times. Hearts and lungs need to be transplanted within 4–6 hours from recovery, liver about 8–10 hours and pancreas about 15 hours; kidneys are the most resilient to ischemia. Kidneys packaged on ice can be successfully transplanted 24–36 hours after recovery. Developments in kidney preservation have yielded a device that pumps cold preservation solution through the kidneys vessels to prevent Delayed Graft Function (DGF) due to ischemia. Perfusion devices, often called kidney pumps, can extend graft survival to 36–48 hours post recovery for kidneys. Research and development is currently underway for heart and lung preservation devices, in an effort to increase distances procurement teams may travel to recover an organ.

2.15.8   Suicide

People committing suicide have a higher rate of donating organs than average. One reason is lower negative response or refusal rate by the family and relatives, but the explanation for this remains to be clarified.[109] In addition, donation consent is higher than average from people committing suicide.[110]

Attempted suicide is a common cause of brain death (3.8%), mainly among young men.[109] Organ donation is more common in this group compared to other causes of death. Brain death may result in legal death, but still with the heart beating, and with mechanical ventilation all other vital organs may be kept completely alive and functional,[70] providing optimal opportunities for organ transplantation.

2.15.9   Controversies

In 2008, California transplant surgeon Hootan Roozrokh was charged with dependent adult abuse for prescribing what prosecutors alleged were excessive doses of morphine and sedatives to hasten the death of a man with adrenal leukodystrophy and irreversible brain damage, in order to procure his organs for transplant.[111] The case brought against Roozrokh was the first criminal case against a transplant surgeon in the US, and resulted in his acquittal.

At California's Emanuel Medical Center, neurologist Narges Pazouki, MD, said an organ-procurement organization representative pressed her to declare a patient brain-dead before the appropriate tests had been done.[107]

In September 1999, eBay blocked an auction for "one functional human kidney" which had reached a highest bid of

$5.7 million. Under United States federal laws, eBay was obligated to dismiss the auction for the selling of human organs which is punishable by up to five years in prison and a $50,000 fine.[112]

On June 27, 2008, Indonesian Sulaiman Damanik, 26, pleaded guilty in a Singapore court for sale of his kidney to CK Tang's executive chair, Mr. Tang Wee Sung, 55, for 150 million rupiah (US$17,000). The Transplant Ethics Committee must approve living donor kidney transplants. Organ trading is banned in Singapore and in many other countries to prevent the exploitation of "poor and socially disadvantaged donors who are unable to make informed choices and suffer potential medical risks." Toni, 27, the other accused, donated a kidney to an Indonesian patient in March, alleging he was the patient's adopted son, and was paid 186 million rupiah (US$21,000).

2.15.10   Social media

The United States Department of Health funded a study by the University of Wisconsin Hospital to increase efforts to increase awareness and the amount of registered donors by pursuing members of the university and their family and friends through social media.[113] The results of the study showed a 20% increase in organ donation by creating support and awareness through social media.[113]

2.15.11   Becoming a donor

Adding one's name to a statewide organ donor registry is the recommended method for ensuring the decision to become an organ, eye and tissue donor is honored. Methods to join the donor registry vary somewhat by state. The most common way to register is through the DMV (Department of Motor Vehicles) or similar agency, typically when renewing a driver's license or ID card.

Alternately, most states also have online portals to their donor registries, which can be accessed through Donate Life America or the U.S. Department of Health and Human Services.

Sharing one's decision to donate with family members is very important, also. Although most states honor First Person Authorization (through donor registries, signing the back of a driver's license, living wills, etc.), the family's cooperation is vital in order to obtain medical and social background information to help determine the health of the donor's organs and tissues. Family challenges to the donor's legally documented decision to donate can cause delays, and may mean fewer organs can be transplanted as the organs deteriorate in the time after death is declared. To be considered as a living organ donor a person should contact a hospital with a transplant center/program. If the desire is to donate to a particular patient, then that patient's transplant center is the one which should be contacted. A list of transplant centers can be found through the Organ Procurement and Transplantation Network.

In the United Kingdom, one signs up to be an organ donor through the NHS Blood and Transplant Service, or on an application for a driving license. This is shown on the photocard part of the license as a code (115).[114]

2.15.12   Public service announcements

There is a need for more participants in organ donation. Marketing for organ donation must walk a fine line between stressing the need for organ donation and not being too forceful.[115] If the marketing agent is too forceful, then the target of the message will react defensively to the request. According to psychological reactance theory, a person will perceive their freedom threatened and will react to restore the freedom. According to Ashley Anker, the use of transportation theory has a positive effect on target reactions by marketing attempts.[115] When public service announcements use recipient-focused messages, targets were more transported. Individuals who watched recipient-focused messages were more transported because potential donors experience empathy for the potential recipient. Future public service announcements should use recipient-focused stories to elicit relationship formation between potential donors and recipients.

Awareness about organ donation leads to greater social support for organ donation, in turn leading to greater registration. By starting with promoting college students' awareness of organ donation and moving to increasing social support for organ donation, the more likely people will be to register as organ donors.[116]

Shortages

Currently more than 100,000 people are waiting for an organ transplant, yet there is a shortage of donors. Over the years people all over the world have stopped registering to be organ donors, resulting in the deaths of numerous people each year. The shortage often creates unethical situations where payments are made in return for the sale of the organs and donors often do not receive appropriate postoperative care. Although most organs may only be taken from donors that have been declared dead (brain-dead), kidneys have remained an exception with their potential for live donor transplants and as such are often the target of illegal harvesting and black market transactions. Many countries have now started to move towards a system of donation by default on death ("Opt Out" system) unless a signed objection is registered with the relevant authorities in order to relieve the burden being placed on the health care system at the moment.

2.15.13   See also

- Australian Organ Donor Register

- Organ transplantation in Israel

- Organ transplantation in China

- MOHAN Foundation

- Sri Lanka Eye Donation Society

- Donate Life America

2.15.14   References

[1] Weaver, Matthew (23 April 2015). "Parents of UK's youngest organ donor hope others will be inspired". *The Guardian* (London). Retrieved 2015-04-24.

[2] http://www.cbsnews.com/news/ growing-human-kidneys-in-rats-sparks-ethical-debate/

[3] http://onlinelibrary.wiley.com/doi/10.1111/ajt.13149/ abstract

[4] Johnson, Eric J.; Goldstein, Daniel G. (21 November 2003). "Do defaults save lives?" (PDF). *Science* **302** (5649): 1338–9. doi:10.1126/science.1091721. PMID 14631022. Retrieved 2012-05-19.

[5] Thaler, Richard H. (September 26, 2009). "Opting in vs. Opting Out". *The New York Times*. Archived from the original on March 8, 2014. Retrieved March 7, 2014.

[6] "Myth busting". *DonateLife*. Australian Government Organ and Tissue Authority. My family can overrule my decision to be a donor. Archived from the original on 22 May 2013. Retrieved 15 May 2013.

[7] http://www.thelocal.es/20150113/ spain-tops-world-organ-transplant-rankings

[8] Organ Donation Taskforce (2008). "The potential impact of an opt out system for organ donation in the UK" (PDF). United Kingdom: Department of Health. p. 22. Retrieved 8 March 2014.

[9] D'Alessandro, Anthony; Peltier, James; Dahl, Andrew (27 November 2012). "Use of social media and college student organizations to increase support for organ donation and advocacy: a case report". *Progress in Transplantation* **22** (4): 436–41. doi:10.7182/pit2012920. PMID 23187063.

[10] Siminoff, Laura; Agyemang, Amma; Traino, Heather (28 February 2013). "Consent to organ donation: a review". *Progress in Transplantation*.   doi:10.7182/pit2013801. PMID 23448829.

[11] "Organ Procurement and Transplantation Network". *http://optn.transplant.hrsa.gov/*. U.S. Department of Health & Human Services. Retrieved 11 October 2015.

[12] "Need continues to grow". *http://optn.transplant.hrsa.gov/*. U.S. Department of Health & Human Services. Retrieved 11 October 2015.

[13] Orentlicher, David (2009). "Presumed Consent to Organ Donation: Its Rise and Fall in the United States" (PDF). *Rutgers Law Review* **61** (2): 295–331.

[14] Tabarrok, Alex (January 8, 2010). "The Meat Market". The Saturday Essay. *The Wall Street Journal*.

[15] Carney, Scott. "The Case for Mandatory Organ Donation". *Wired*. Conde Naste. Retrieved 13 February 2015.

[16] Wiggins, Ovetta. "Pa. organ donors get $300 boost It pays for food or lodging for them or their family. A bigger plan's rejection rankles some.". *Philly.com*. Philadelphia Media Network. Retrieved 28 February 2015.

[17] Krauthammer, Charles. "Yes, Let's Pay for Organs". *Time*. Time Inc. Retrieved 28 February 2015.

[18] Gormley, Michael (April 27, 2010). "New York To Be First Organ Donor Opt-Out State?". New York. *The Huffington Post* (New York City). Archived from the original on April 30, 2010. Retrieved March 7, 2014.

[19] "Organ donation opt-out system given go-ahead in Wales". BBC News. July 2, 2013. Archived from the original on March 7, 2014. Retrieved March 7, 2014.

[20] "MEPs back Europe organ donor card". BBC News. 22 April 2008. Archived from the original on 2 August 2012. Retrieved 8 March 2014.

[21] "Come donare" [How to Donate] (in Italian). Ministry of Health (Italy). Archived from the original on 8 March 2014. Retrieved 13 January 2013.

[22] Jones, Meg (23 April 2011). "A Soldier's Death Gives Life to Another Man". United States: Pulitzer Center on Crisis Reporting. Archived from the original on 26 August 2013. Retrieved 8 March 2014.

[23] Wicks, Mona Newsome (25 April 2000). "Brain Death and Transplantation: The Japanese". *Medscape Transplantation* (Medscape). Retrieved 8 March 2014.

[24] Vyas, Hetel (January 14, 2013). "State goes slow on stiffer jail term for organ scamsters". *The Times of India*. Archived from the original on March 7, 2014. Retrieved March 7, 2014.

[25] Kurup, Deepa (January 4, 2013). "Expendable cogs in a well-oiled racket". *The Hindu* (India). Archived from the original on March 10, 2013. Retrieved March 7, 2014.

[26] "Govt amends Transplantation of Human Organs Act". *Zee News* (India). March 17, 2011. Archived from the original on March 7, 2014. Retrieved March 7, 2014.

[27] "National Workshop of transplant coordinators provides guidelines". *The Hindu* (India). March 7, 2013. Archived from the original on May 11, 2013. Retrieved March 7, 2014.

[28] Dhar, Aarti (19 December 2009). "Organ Transplant Bill tabled". *The Hindu*. Archived from the original on 8 March 2014. Retrieved 8 March 2014.

[29] *The Transplantation of Human Organs (Amendment) Bill, 2011*, Act No. 136-C of 2009. Retrieved on 8 March 2014.

[30] Sreeraman (23 November 2009). "Amendments in Transplantation of Human Organ Act, 1994". *Medindia*. Archived from the original on 8 March 2014. Retrieved 8 March 2014.

[31] Shroff, Sunil (Jul–Sep 2009). "Legal and ethical aspects of organ donation and transplantation". *Indian J. Urol.* **25** (3): 348–55. doi:10.4103/0970-1591.56203. PMC 2779960. PMID 19881131.

[32] Shroff, Sunil (2009). "Organ Donation and Transplantation in India – Legal Aspects & Solutions to Help With Shortage of Organs". *J. Nephrol. Ren. Transplant.* **2** (1): 23–34. ISSN 1918-0268.

[33] "Illegal organ transplant can attract 10-year jail". *The Hindu*. 13 August 2011. Archived from the original on 8 March 2014. Retrieved 8 March 2014.

[34] "Ann 4 THOA ACT 2011" (PDF). Organ Retrieval Banking Organization. Archived (PDF) from the original on 8 March 2014. Retrieved 8 March 2014.

[35] "Lok Sabha approves tougher organ transplant Bill". *India Today*. 13 August 2011. Archived from the original on 21 August 2013.

[36] "RS seal on amendment to human organs bill". *The Times of India*. 27 August 2011.

[37] Express News Service (August 13, 2011). "LS okays amendments to organ transplantation Bill". Archive. *The Indian Express* (India). Archived from the original on March 7, 2014. Retrieved March 7, 2014.

[38] Kannan, Ramya (22 January 2002). "Organ donation gains momentum". Southern States. *The Hindu* (India). Archived from the original on 8 March 2014. Retrieved 8 March 2014.

[39] Kannan, Ramya (28 February 2003). "High time to streamline organ transplants". Southern States. *The Hindu* (India). Archived from the original on 13 December 2013. Retrieved 8 March 2014.

[40] Raman, Usha (25 July 2002). "Living after death". Metro Plus Hyderabad. *The Hindu* (India). Archived from the original on 29 November 2010. Retrieved 8 March 2014.

[41] Joseph, Lison (28 January 2004). "Organ transplantation help at hand". Hyderabad. *The Times of India*. Retrieved 8 March 2014.

[42] "Cadaveric Organ Donation Figures". MOHAN Foundation. INOS Figures (2000 - 2009). Archived from the original on 2 January 2014. Retrieved 8 March 2014.

[43] Navin, Sumana (2008). "Government Orders on Organ Donation and Transplantation From Tamil Nadu Health Department". MOHAN Foundation. Archived from the original on 11 December 2013. Retrieved 8 March 2014.

[44] Srinivasan, Sandhya (2013). "Has Tamil Nadu turned the tide on the transplant trade?". *BMJ* (United Kingdom) **346**: f2155. doi:10.1136/bmj.f2155. PMID 23585066.

[45] Reddy, Sunil K. Vemuru; et al. (January–March 2011). "Live related donors in India: Their quality of life using world health organization quality of life brief questionnaire". *Indian J. Urol.* **27** (1): 25–9. doi:10.4103/0970-1591.78411. PMC 3114583. PMID 21716885.

[46] "Sri Lanka donates eyes to the world". *Foxnews.com*. Associated Press. 23 January 2012. Archived from the original on 23 January 2014. Retrieved 9 March 2014.

[47] Carneiro, Julia (1 June 2014). "How thousands of football fans are helping to save lives". *BBC News Magazine*.

[48] Organ Donation New Zealand "Number of transplant operations in New Zealand" http://www.donor.co.nz/statistics/number-of-transplant-operations-in-new-zealand

[49] "Human Tissue Act 2008". New Zealand Legislature. 1 July 2013. Public Act 2008 No 28. Retrieved 2015-08-10.

[50] "Number of deceased organ donors in New Zealand". *Statistics*. Organ Donation New Zealand. Archived from the original on 30 May 2014.

[51] "Organ and tissue donation". *Getting a license*. NZ Transport Agency.

[52] "Kidney Donation". *Nephrology Department, Christchurch Hospital, New Zealand*. Canterbury District Health Board. October 2011. Archived from the original on 29 November 2014.

[53] New Zealand Parliament "Human Tissue (Organ Donation) Amendment Bill" http://www.parliament.nz/en-nz/pb/legislation/bills/00DBHOH_BILL7223_1/human-tissue-organ-donation-amendment-bill

[54] New Zealand Herald. "Doctors oppose organ donor bill" http://www.nzherald.co.nz/nz/news/article.cfm?c_id=1&objectid=10379728

[55] Mauri Ora Associates Limited. "Māori Pacific Attitudes Towards Transplantation: Professional Perspectives" https://www.health.govt.nz/system/files/documents/pages/maori-pacific-attitudes-towards-transplantation.pdf

[56] Ghods, Ahad J.; Savaj, Shekoufeh (November 2006). "Iranian Model of Paid and Regulated Living-Unrelated Kidney Donation". *Clinical Journal of the American Society of Nephrology*. doi:10.2215/CJN.00700206. PMID 17699338.

[57] Easterbrook, Gregg. "Organ Donation: Where Your Religion Stands". *BeliefNet*. Archived from the original on 10 November 2013. Retrieved 9 March 2014. Despite popular misconceptions, there are almost no religious rules against donating organs or receiving transplants. A few denominations ban these practices, and a few others have rules that are not models of clarity. *This is the first of two pages.*

[58] Zargooshi, Javaad (2001). "Quality of life of Iranian kidney "donors"". *J. Urol.* **166** (5): 1790–9. doi:10.1016/S0022-5347(05)65677-7. PMID 11586226.

[59] Goyal, Madhav; et al. (2002). "Economic and health consequences of selling a kidney in India". *JAMA* **288** (13): 1589–93. doi:10.1001/jama.288.13.1589. PMID 12350189.

[60] Sidner, Sara; Eastment, Tess (29 January 2008). "Police hunt for doctor in kidney-snatching ring". CNN. Archived from the original on 9 November 2012. Retrieved 8 March 2014.

[61] Matas, David; Kilgour, David (31 January 2007). "Bloody Harvest: Report into Allegations of Organ Harvesting of Falun Gong Practitioners in China" (PDF). Archived (PDF) from the original on 15 February 2014. Retrieved 8 March 2014.

[62] Adams, David (27 May 2003). "Organ trafficking suspected in mass murder case". *The Times* (United Kingdom). Retrieved 8 March 2014.

[63] Kelly, Annie (September 6, 2009). "Child sacrifice and ritual murder rise as famine looms". *The Guardian* (London). Archived from the original on February 14, 2014. Retrieved March 7, 2014.

[64] Carney, Scott (8 May 2007). "Why a Kidney (Street Value: $3,000) Sells for $85,000". *Wired*. Archived from the original on 29 July 2013. Retrieved 8 March 2014.

[65] Jan, Sadaqat (12 November 2006). "Poor Pakistanis Donate Kidneys for Money". *The Washington Post*. Associated Press. Retrieved 8 March 2014.

[66] Sarvestani, Nima (31 October 2006). "Iran's desperate kidney traders". BBC News. Archived from the original on 13 November 2013. Retrieved 8 March 2014.

[67] Carney, Scott (8 May 2007). "Inside 'Kidneyville': Rani's Story". *Wired*. Archived from the original on 23 June 2013. Retrieved 8 March 2014.

[68] Scheper-Hughes, Nancy. "The new cannibalism". *Berkeley Digital Library SunSITE*. University of California, Berkeley. Archived from the original on 3 May 2009.

[69] Stix, Gary (4 January 2011). "Donate Your Brain, Save a Buck". *Scientific American* **304** (1): 29. Retrieved 8 March 2014.

[70] Heisler, Jennifer (29 June 2013). "Organ Donation After Brain Death". *About.com*. Retrieved 9 March 2014.

[71] Sanford, John; Dubois, Gèrard (Spring 2011). "When Are You Dead?". *Stanford Medicine Magazine* **28** (1). United States: Stanford University School of Medicine. Archived from the original on 15 November 2013. Retrieved 9 March 2014.

[72] Bird, Shiela M.; Harris, John (2010). "Time to move to presumed consent for organ donation". Analysis. *BMJ* **340**: c2188. doi:10.1136/bmj.c2188. PMID 20442244.

[73] R.M. (anonymous) (7 December 2011). "Organ sales: Paying to live" (blog). *The Economist*. London. Archived from the original on 19 June 2013. Retrieved 9 March 2014. Iran adopted a system of paying kidney donors in 1988 and within 11 years it became the only country in the world to clear its waiting list for transplants.

[74] Appel, Jacob (May–June 2005). "Organ Solicitation on the Internet: Every Man for Himself?". *Hastings Cent. Rep.* **35** (3): 14–15. doi:10.1353/hcr.2005.0052. PMID 16092393.

[75] "Trasplantes" [Transplants] (in Spanish). Spain: National Transplant Organization. Los españoles, un ejemplo imitado. Archived from the original on 6 January 2014. Retrieved 9 March 2014.

[76] Archived March 8, 2014 at the Wayback Machine

[77] "More countries hope to copy Spain's organ-donation success". Canadian Medical Association. 29 September 2003. Archived from the original on August 28, 2009. Retrieved 2011-03-31.

[78] Estelle v Gamble 429 U.S. 97, 97 S. Ct. 285 50l Ed 2d251 [1976]

[79] "U.S. Statement On Prison Status and Organ Allocation". United Network for Organ Sharing. 2002-06-02. Archived from the original on September 26, 2006. Retrieved 2009-12-20.

[80] Wiegand, Steve (January 25, 2002). "State inmate gets new heart; 'Medically necessary care' is required by law, an official says". *The Sacramento Bee*.

[81] Ingalls, Chris (8 April 2005). "Prison inmate awaits organ transplant" (PDF). *KING-TV*. Association of Washington Cities. Archived from the original (PDF) on 6 January 2009. Retrieved 20 December 2009.

[82] Attack of the Clones...And the Issue of the Clones, 3 Colum. Paul Lesko and Kevin Buckley – Sci. & Tech L. Rev. 1, 19 (2002)

[83] Killer in Need of a Kidney Starts Ethics Row, Lee Douglas – Chicago Tribune, May 29, 2003, at 10.

[84] Perry, David L. "Should Violent Felons Receive Organ Transplants?". Markkula Center for Applied Ethics. Retrieved 2009-12-20.

[85] Guidelines for Preventing HIV Through Transplantation of Human Tissue and Organs, CDC Recommendations and Reports, May 20, 1994 /43(RR-8); 1–17.

[86] O'Reilly, Kevin B. (9 April 2007). "Prisoner organ donation proposal worrisome". *American Medical News*. Archived from the original on 30 September 2013. Retrieved 8 March 2014.

[87] http://www.gavelife.org – Organization established to advocate for organ donations from prisoners.

[88] "Sheriff Teaches Inmates to "Have a Heart" By Volunteering To Give Up Theirs". Committee to Re-Elect Joe Arpaio 2008. 13 June 2007. Archived from the original on 14 January 2009. Retrieved 20 October 2008.

[89] http://www.msco.org – See Maricopa County's "I DO" program.

[90] "Inside the Kidney Cult". *The Sydney Morning Herald*. 30 March 2008. Archived from the original on 17 April 2012. Retrieved 8 March 2014.

[91] "(untitled)" (Microsoft PowerPoint). *Give and Let Live*. United Kingdom: NHS Blood and Transplant. Archived from the original on 8 March 2014. Retrieved 8 March 2014.

[92] "Statements from Religions". American Red Cross. Jehovah's Witness. Archived from the original on 17 September 2008. Retrieved 22 July 2008.

[93] "Shinto: Organ donation". BBC. 16 September 2009. Archived from the original on 29 December 2013. Retrieved 8 March 2014.

[94] Sinclair 2003, p.242

[95] "UNOS", United Network for Organ Sharing. Transplant Trends. Retrieved 8 March 2014. Waiting list candidates as of today 2:24pm

[96] Stein, Rob (22 March 2008). "A Third of Patients On The Transplant List Are Not Eligible". *The Washington Post*. Retrieved 8 March 2014.

[97] "Resources - General Public". California Transplant Donor Network. Waiting List Statistics. Archived from the original on 19 August 2010. Retrieved 2011-03-31.

[98] "OHSU Transplant Program". Oregon Health & Science University. 16 March 2011. Retrieved 31 March 2011. *Link redirects to page without the required information; original page has been excluded from Internet Archive.*

[99] "Organ & Tissue Donation Western Australia (WA)" (PDF). DonateLife in Western Australia. Archived from the original (PDF) on September 27, 2007. Retrieved 2011-03-31.

[100] "Lions Eye Institute: Lions Eye Bank". Lei.org.au. 2011-06-30. Retrieved 2012-05-19.

[101] Dubner, Stephen J.; Levitt, Steven D. (2006-07-09). "Flesh Trade". New York Times.

[102] Thaler, Richard H. (2009-09-26). "Opting In vs. Opting Out". New York Times.

[103] Ghods AJ, Savaj S (2006). "Iranian model of paid and regulated living-unrelated kidney donation". *Clin J Am Soc Nephrol* **1** (6): 1136–45. doi:10.2215/CJN.00700206. PMID 17699338.

[104] "Financial Incentives for Organ Donation". Archived from the original on 17 May 2013. *After May 2013, this page was no longer available for archiving; in March 2014, searches of the kidney.org site did not reveal a comparable statement in current online materials.*

[105] "Lifesharers.org".

[106] Richard Schwindt and Aidan Vining (1998). "Proposal for a Mutual Insurance Pool for Transplant Organs". *Journal of Health Politics, Policy and Law* **23** (5): 725–41.

[107] Rob Stein (2007-09-13). "New Zeal in Organ Procurement Raises Fears". *The Washington Post* (The Washington Post Company). Retrieved 2008-05-02.

[108] Solving the Organ Shortage. Center for Ethical Solutions. Retrieved on 2009-07-08. Archived April 13, 2009 at the Wayback Machine

[109] Figueiredo FM, Capaverde FB, Londero GG, et al. (March 2007). "Organ donation in suicides". *Transplant. Proc.* **39** (2): 344–5. doi:10.1016/j.transproceed.2007.01.015. PMID 17362725.

[110] Moraes BN, Bacal F, Teixeira MC, et al. (April 2009). "Behavior profile of family members of donors and non-donors of organs". *Transplant. Proc.* **41** (3): 799–801. doi:10.1016/j.transproceed.2009.02.043. PMID 19376356.

[111] Jesse McKinley (2008-02-27). "Surgeon Accused of Speeding a Death to Get Organs". *The New York Time* (The New York Times Company). Retrieved 2008-05-02.

[112] J.H. Huebert (1999-09-24). "Human Organs and Ebay: A Combination That Could Save Lives". *The Collegian*. Archived from the original on July 7, 2007. Retrieved 2009-11-17.

[113] Peltier, James W., Anthony M. Allessandro, and Andrew J. Dahl. "Use of Social Media and College Student Organizations to Increase Support for Organ Donation and Advocacy: A Case Report." Progress in Transplantation (2012): 436-41.

[114] Gov.uk, Driving license codes, https://www.gov.uk/driving-licence-codes

[115] Reinhart, A. M. and A. E. Anker (2012). "An Exploration of Transportation and Psychological Reactance in Organ Donation PSAs." Communication Research Reports 29(4): 274-284.

[116] Feeley, TH, Peltier, JW, D'Alessandro, AM, Dahl, AJ (2013). "A sequential decision framework for increasing college students' support for organ donation and organ donor registration". *Progress in Transplantation*.

2.15.15   External links

- National Institute of Health's MedLine on Organ Donation

- UK Transplant, part of NHS Blood and Transplant

- OrganDonor.gov (USA)

- Portal for Organ Donation After Execution

- Portal for The National Network of Organ Donors

- Human Tissue Donation – NPR News Investigation

- G.A.V.E Life Prisoner Organ Donation

- Organ and Tissue Donation What Every Nurse Needs to Know course on www.RN.org

2.16   Persistent vegetative state

A **persistent vegetative state** is a disorder of consciousness in which patients with severe brain damage are in a state of partial arousal rather than true awareness. It is a diagnosis of some uncertainty in that it deals with a syndrome. After four weeks in a **vegetative state** (VS), the patient is classified as in a persistent (or 'continuing') vegetative state. This diagnosis is classified as a **permanent vegetative state** (PVS) some months after a non-traumatic brain injury (3 months in the US, 6 months in the UK, or one year after traumatic injury). Nowadays, more doctors and (neuro)scientists prefer to call the state of consciousness an **unresponsive wakefulness syndrome**, primarily because of ethical questions about whether a patient can be called 'vegetative' or not. [1]

2.16.1   Definition

There are several definitions that vary by technical versus laymen's usage. There are different legal implications in different countries.

Medical definition

A wakeful unconscious state that lasts longer than a few weeks is referred to as a persistent (or 'continuing') vegetative state.[2][3]

Lack of legal clarity

Unlike brain death, permanent vegetative state (PVS) is recognized by *statute law* as death in very few legal systems. In the US, courts have required petitions before termination of life support that demonstrate that any recovery of cognitive functions above a vegetative state is assessed as impossible by authoritative medical opinion.[4] In England and Wales the legal precedent for withdrawal of clinically assisted nutrition and hydration in cases of patients in a PVS was set in 1993 in the case of Tony Bland, who sustained catastrophic anoxic brain injury in the 1989 Hillsborough disaster.[2] Application to the Court of Protection is still now required before nutrition and hydration can be withdrawn or withheld from PVS (or 'minimally conscious' - MCS) patients.[5]

This legal grey area has led to vocal advocates that those in PVS should be allowed to die. Others are equally determined that, if recovery is at all possible, care should continue. The existence of a small number of diagnosed PVS cases that have eventually resulted in improvement makes defining recovery as "impossible" particularly difficult in a legal sense.[6] This legal and ethical issue raises questions about autonomy, quality of life, appropriate use of resources, the wishes of family members, and professional responsibilities.

Vegetative state

The vegetative state is a chronic or long-term condition. This condition differs from a coma: a coma is a state that lacks both awareness and wakefulness. Patients in a vegetative state may have awoken from a coma, but still have not regained awareness. In the vegetative state patients can open their eyelids occasionally and demonstrate sleep-wake cycles, but completely lack cognitive function. The vegetative state is also called a "coma vigil". The chances of regaining awareness diminish considerably as the time spent in the vegetative state increases.[7]

Persistent vegetative state

Persistent vegetative state is the standard usage (except in the UK) for a medical diagnosis, made after numerous neurological and other tests, that due to extensive and irrevocable brain damage a patient is *highly unlikely* ever to achieve higher functions above a vegetative state. This diagnosis does not mean that a doctor has diagnosed improvement as impossible, but does open the possibility, in the US, for a judicial request to end life support.[6] Informal guidelines hold that this diagnosis can be made after four weeks in a vegetative state. US caselaw has shown that successful petitions for termination have been made after a diagnosis of a persistent vegetative state, although in some cases, such as that of Terri Schiavo, such rulings have generated widespread controversy.

In the UK, the term 'persistent vegetative state' is discouraged in favor of two more precisely defined terms that have been strongly recommended by the Royal College of Physicians (RCP). These guidelines recommend using a **continuous vegetative state** for patients in a vegetative state for more than four weeks. A medical definition of a **permanent vegetative state** can be made if, after exhaustive testing and a customary 12 months of observation,[8] a medical diagnosis that it is *impossible* by any informed medical expectations that the mental condition will ever improve.[9] Hence, a "continuous vegetative state" in the UK may remain the diagnosis in cases that would be called "persistent" in the US or elsewhere.

While the actual testing criteria for a diagnosis of "permanent" in the UK are quite similar to the criteria for a diagnosis of "persistent" in the US, the semantic difference imparts in the UK a *legal* presumption that is commonly used in court applications for ending life support.[8] The UK diagnosis is generally only made after 12 months of observing a static vegetative state. A diagnosis of a persistent vegetative state in the US usually still requires a petitioner to prove in court that recovery is impossible by informed medical opinion, while in the UK the "permanent" diagnosis already gives the petitioner this presumption and may make the legal process less time-consuming.[6]

In common usage, the "permanent" and "persistent" definitions are sometimes conflated and used interchangeably. However, the acronym "PVS" is intended to define a "persistent vegetative state", without necessarily the connotations of permanence, and is used as such throughout this article.

Bryan Jennett, who originally coined the term "persistent vegetative state", has now recommended using the UK division between continuous and permanent in his most recent book *The Vegetative State*. This is one for purposes of precision, on the grounds that "the 'persistent' component of this term ... may seem to suggest irreversibility".[10]

The Australian National Health and Medical Research Council has suggested "post coma unresponsiveness" as an alternative term for "vegetative state" in general.[11]

2.16.2 Signs and symptoms

Most PVS patients are unresponsive to external stimuli and their conditions are associated with different levels of consciousness. Some level of consciousness means a person can still respond, in varying degrees, to stimulation. A person in a coma, however, cannot. In addition, PVS patients often open their eyes in response to feeding, which has to be done by others; they are capable of swallowing, whereas patients in a coma subsist with their eyes closed (Emmett, 1989).

PVS patients' eyes might be in a relatively fixed position, or track moving objects, or move in a *disconjugate* (i.e., completely unsynchronized) manner. They may experience sleep-wake cycles, or be in a state of chronic wakefulness. They may exhibit some behaviors that can be construed as arising from partial consciousness, such as grinding their teeth, swallowing, smiling, shedding tears, grunting, moaning, or screaming without any apparent external stimulus.

Individuals in PVS are seldom on any life-sustaining equipment other than a feeding tube because the brainstem, the center of vegetative functions (such as heart rate and rhythm, respiration, and gastrointestinal activity) is relatively intact (Emmett, 1989).

Recovery

Many people emerge spontaneously from a vegetative state within a few weeks.[10] The chances of recovery depend on the extent of injury to the brain and the patient's age – younger patients having a better chance of recovery than older patients. A 1994 report found that of those who were in a vegetative state a month after a trauma, 54% had regained consciousness by a year after the trauma, whereas 28% had died and 18% were still in the vegetative state. But for non-traumatic injuries such as strokes, only 14% had recovered consciousness at one year, 47% had died, and 39% were still vegetative. Patients who were vegetative six months after the initial event were much less likely to have recovered consciousness a year after the event than in the case of those who were simply reported vegetative at one month.[12] A New Scientist article from 2000 gives a pair of graphs showing changes of patient status during the first 12 months after head injury and after incidents depriving the brain of oxygen.[13] After a year, the chances that a PVS patient will regain consciousness are very low[14] and most patients who do recover consciousness experience significant disability. The longer a patient is in a PVS, the more severe the resulting disabilities are likely to be. Rehabilitation can contribute to recovery, but many patients never progress to the point of being able to take care of themselves. Recovery after long periods of time in a PVS has been reported on several occasions and is often treated as a spectacular event.

There are two dimensions of recovery from a persistent vegetative state: recovery of consciousness and recovery of function. Recovery of consciousness can be verified by reliable evidence of awareness of self and the environment, consistent voluntary behavioral responses to visual and auditory stimuli, and interaction with others. Recovery of function is characterized by communication, the ability to learn and to perform adaptive tasks, mobility, self-care, and participation in recreational or vocational activities. Recovery of consciousness may occur without functional recovery, but functional recovery cannot occur without recovery of consciousness (Ashwal, 1994).

2.16.3 Causes

There are three main causes of PVS (persistent vegetative state):

1. Acute traumatic brain injury

2. Non-traumatic: neurodegenerative disorder or metabolic disorder of the brain

3. Severe congenital abnormality of the central nervous system

Medical books (such as Lippincott, Williams, and Wilkins. (2007). In A Page: Pediatric Signs and Symptoms) describe several potential causes of PVS, which are as follows:

- Bacterial, viral, or fungal infection, including meningitis

- Increased intracranial pressure, such as a tumor or abscess

- Vascular pressure which causes intracranial hemorrhaging or stroke

- Hypoxic ischemic injury (hypotension, cardiac arrest, arrhythmia, near-drowning)

- Toxins such as uremia, ethanol, atropine, opiates, lead, colloidal silver[15]

- Trauma: Concussion, contusion

- Seizure, both nonconvulsive status epilepticus and postconvulsive state (postictal state)

- Electrolyte imbalance, which involves hyponatremia, hypernatremia, hypomagnesemia, hypoglycemia, hyperglycemia, hypercalcemia, and hypocalcemia

- Postinfectious: Acute disseminated encephalomyelitis (ADEM)

- Endocrine disorders such as adrenal insufficiency and thyroid disorders

- Degenerative and metabolic diseases including urea cycle disorders, Reye syndrome, and mitochondrial disease

- Systemic infection and sepsis

- Hepatic encephalopathy

In addition, these authors claim that doctors sometimes use the mnemonic device AEIOU-TIPS to recall portions of the differential diagnosis: Alcohol ingestion and acidosis, Epilepsy and encephalopathy, Infection, Opiates, Uremia, Trauma, Insulin overdose or inflammatory disorders, Poisoning and psychogenic causes, and Shock.

2.16.4 Diagnosis

Despite converging agreement about the definition of persistent vegetative state, recent reports have raised concerns about the accuracy of diagnosis in some patients, and the extent to which, in a selection of cases, residual cognitive functions may remain undetected and patients are diagnosed as being in a persistent vegetative state. Objective assessment of residual cognitive function can be extremely difficult as motor responses may be minimal, inconsistent, and difficult to document in many patients, or may be undetectable in others because no cognitive output is possible (Owen et al, 2002). In recent years, a number of studies have demonstrated an important role for functional neuroimaging in the identification of residual cognitive function in persistent vegetative state; this technology is providing new insights into cerebral activity in patients with severe brain damage. Such studies, when successful, may be particularly useful where there is concern about the accuracy of the diagnosis and the possibility that residual cognitive function has remained undetected.

Diagnostic experiments

Researchers have begun to use functional neuroimaging studies to study implicit cognitive processing in patients with a clinical diagnosis of persistent vegetative state. Activations in response to sensory stimuli with positron emission tomography (PET), functional magnetic resonance imaging (fMRI), and electrophysiological methods can provide information on the presence, degree, and location of any residual brain function. However, use of these techniques in people with severe brain damage is methodologically, clinically, and theoretically complex and needs careful quantitative analysis and interpretation.

For example, PET studies have shown the identification of residual cognitive function in persistent vegetative state. That is, an external stimulation, such as a painful stimulus, still activates 'primary' sensory cortices in these patients but these areas are functionally disconnected from 'higher order' associative areas needed for awareness. These results show that parts of the cortex are indeed still functioning in 'vegetative' patients (Matsuda et al, 2003).

In addition, other PET studies have revealed preserved and consistent responses in predicted regions of auditory cortex in response to intelligible speech stimuli. Moreover, a preliminary fMRI examination revealed partially intact responses to semantically ambiguous stimuli, which are known to tap higher aspects of speech comprehension (Boly, 2004).

Furthermore, several studies have used PET to assess the central processing of noxious somatosensory stimuli in patients in PVS. Noxious somatosensory stimulation activated midbrain, contralateral thalamus, and primary somatosensory cortex in each and every PVS patient, even in the absence of detectable cortical evoked potentials. In conclusion, somatosensory stimulation of PVS patients, at intensities that elicited pain in controls, resulted in increased neuronal activity in primary somatosensory cortex, even if resting brain metabolism was severely impaired. However, this activation of primary cortex seems to be isolated and dissociated from higher-order associative cortices (Laureys et al, 2002).

Also, there is evidence of partially functional cerebral regions in catastrophically injured brains. To study five patients in PVS with different behavioral features, researchers employed PET, MRI and magnetoencephalographic (MEG) responses to sensory stimulation. In three of the five patients, co-registered PET/MRI correlate areas of relatively preserved brain metabolism with isolated fragments of behavior. Two patients had suffered anoxic injuries and demonstrated marked decreases in overall cerebral metabolism to 30–40% of normal. Two other patients with non-anoxic, multifocal brain injuries demonstrated several isolated brain regions with higher metabolic rates, that ranged up to 50–80% of normal. Nevertheless, their global metabolic rates remained <50% of normal. MEG recordings from three PVS patients provide clear evidence for the absence, abnormality or reduction of evoked responses. Despite major abnormalities, however, these data also provide evidence for localized residual activity at the cortical level. Each patient partially preserved restricted sensory representations, as evidenced by slow evoked magnetic fields and gamma band activity. In two patients, these activations correlate with isolated behavioral patterns and metabolic activity. Remaining active regions identified in the three PVS patients with behavioral fragments appear to consist of segregated corticothalamic networks that retain connectivity and partial functional integrity. A single patient who suffered severe injury to the tegmental mesencephalon and paramedian thalamus showed widely preserved cortical metabolism, and a global average metabolic rate of 65% of normal. The relatively high preservation of cortical metabolism in this patient defines the first functional correlate of clinical– pathological reports associating permanent unconsciousness with structural damage to these regions. The specific patterns of preserved metabolic activity identified in these patients reflect novel evidence of the modular nature of individual functional networks that underlie conscious brain function. The variations in cerebral metabolism in chronic PVS patients indicate that some cerebral regions can retain partial function in catastrophically injured brains (Schiff et al, 2002).

Misdiagnoses

Misdiagnosis of PVS is not uncommon. One study of 40 patients in the United Kingdom reported that 43% of those patients classified as in a PVS were misdiagnosed and another 33% able to recover whilst the study was underway.[16] Some cases of PVS may actually be cases of patients being in an undiagnosed minimally conscious state.[17] Since the exact diagnostic criteria of the minimally conscious state were formulated only in 2002, there may be chronic patients diagnosed as PVS before the notion of the minimally conscious state became known.

Whether or not there is conscious awareness in vegetative state is a prominent issue. Three completely different aspects of this issue should be distinguished. First, some patients can be conscious simply because they are misdiagnosed (see above). In fact, they are not in vegetative state. Second, sometimes a patient was correctly diagnosed but, then, examined during a beginning recovery. Third, perhaps some day the very notion of the vegetative state will change so as to include elements of conscious awareness. Inability to disentangle these three cases leads to confusion. An example of such confusion is the response to a recent experiment using functional magnetic resonance imaging which revealed that a woman diagnosed with PVS was able to activate predictable portions of her brain in response to the tester's requests that she imagine herself playing tennis or moving from room to room in her house. The brain activity in response to these instructions was indistinguishable from those of healthy patients.[18][19][20]

In 2010, Martin Monti and fellow researchers, working at the MRC Cognition and Brain Sciences Unit at the University of Cambridge, reported in an article in the New England Journal of Medicine[21] that some patients in persistent vegetative states responded to verbal instructions by displaying different patterns of brain activity on fMRI scans. Five out of a total of 54 diagnosed patients were apparently able to respond when instructed to think about one of two different physical activities. One of these five was also able to "answer" yes or no questions, again by imagining one of these two activities.[22] It is unclear, however, whether the fact that portions of the patients' brains light up on fMRI could help these patients assume their own medical decision making.[22]

In November 2011, a publication in *The Lancet* presented bedside EEG apparatus and indicated that its signal could be used to detect awareness in three of 16 patients diagnosed in the vegetative state.[23]

2.16.5   Treatment

Currently no treatment for vegetative state exists that would satisfy the efficacy criteria of evidence-based medicine. Several methods have been proposed which can roughly be subdivided into four categories: pharmacological methods, surgery, physical therapy, and various stimulation techniques. Pharmacological therapy mainly uses activating substances such as tricyclic antidepressants or methylphenidate. Mixed results have been reported using dopaminergic drugs such as amantadine and bromocriptine and stimulants such as dextroamphetamine.[24] Surgical methods such as deep brain stimulation are used less frequently due to the invasiveness of the procedures. Stimulation techniques include sensory stimulation, sensory regulation, music and musicokinetic therapy, social-tactile interaction, and cortical stimulation.[25]

Zolpidem

There is limited evidence that the hypnotic drug zolpidem has an effect.[26] As of yet, few scientific studies have been published on the effectiveness and the results have been sometimes contradictory.[27][28]

2.16.6   Epidemiology

In the United States, it is estimated that there may be between 15,000–40,000 patients who are in a persistent vegetative state, but due to poor nursing home records exact figures are hard to determine.[29]

2.16.7   History

The syndrome was first described in 1940 by Ernst Kretschmer who called it *apallic syndrome*.[30] The term *persistent vegetative state* was coined in 1972 by Scottish spinal surgeon Bryan Jennett and American neurologist Fred Plum to describe a syndrome that seemed to have been made possible by medicine's increased capacities to keep patients' bodies alive.[10][31]

2.16.8   Society and culture

Ethics and policy

An ongoing debate exists as to how much care, if any, patients in a persistent vegetative state should receive in health systems plagued by limited resources. In a case before the New Jersey Superior Court, *Betancourt v. Trinitas Hospital*, a community hospital sought a ruling that dialysis and CPR for such a patient constitutes futile care. An American bioethicist, Jacob M. Appel, argued that any money spent treating PVS patients would be better spent on other patients with a higher likelihood of recovery.[32] The patient died naturally prior to a decision in the case, resulting in the court finding the issue moot.

In 2010, British and Belgian researchers reported in an article in the *New England Journal of Medicine* that some patients in persistent vegetative states actually had enough consciousness to "answer" yes or no questions on fMRI scans.[33] However, it is unclear whether the fact that portions of the patients' brains light up on fMRI will help these patient assume their own medical decision making.[33] Professor Geraint Rees, Director of the Institute of Cognitive Neuroscience at University College London, responded to the study by observing that, "As a clinician, it would be important to satisfy oneself that the individual that you are communicating with is competent to make those decisions. At the moment it is premature to conclude that the individual able to answer 5 out of 6 yes/no questions is fully conscious like you or I."[33] In contrast, Jacob M. Appel of the Mount Sinai Hospital told the *Telegraph* that this development could be a welcome step toward clarifying the wishes of such patients. Appel stated: "I see no reason why, if we are truly convinced such patients are communicating, society should not honour their wishes. In fact, as a physician, I think a compelling case can be made that doctors have an ethical obligation to assist such patients by removing treatment. I suspect that, if such individuals are indeed trapped in their bodies, they may be living in great torment and will request to have their care terminated or even active euthanasia."[33]

Notable cases

The longest documented case of survival in a persistent vegetative state was Aruna Shanbaug, a nurse in Mumbai, India who remained in persistent vegetative state for 42 years from 1973 to 2015,[34] becoming the longest individual in PVS state until her death.

2.16.9   See also

- Brain death

- Botulism

- Catatonia

- Karolina Olsson

- Locked-in syndrome

- Process Oriented Coma Work, for an approach to working with residual consciousness in patients in comatose and persistent vegetative states

2.16.10   Notes

[1] Laureys S, Celesia GG, Cohadon F, Lavrijsen J, León-Carrión J, Sannita WG, Sazbon L, Schmutzhard E, von Wild KR, Zeman A, Dolce G; European Task Force on Disorders of Consciousness. Unresponsive wakefulness syndrome: a new name for the vegetative state or apallic syndrome. BMC Med. 2010;8(68). doi: 10.1186/1741-7015-8-68

[2] Royal College of Physicians 2013 Prolonged Disorders of Consciousness: National Clinical Guidelines, https://www.rcplondon.ac.uk/resources/prolonged-disorders-consciousness-national-clinical-guidelines

[3] The Multi-Society Task Force on PVS (1994). "Medical Aspects of the Persistent Vegetative State— First of Two Parts". *New England Journal of Medicine* **330** (21): 1499–1508. doi:10.1056/NEJM199405263302107. PMID 7818633.

[4] Jennett, B (1999). "Should cases of permanent vegetative state still go to court?. Britain should follow other countries and keep the courts for cases of dispute". *BMJ (Clinical research ed.)* **319** (7213): 796–97. doi:10.1136/bmj.319.7213.796. PMC 1116645. PMID 10496803.

[5] Royal College of Physicians 2013 Prolonged Disorders of Consciousness: National Clinical Guidelines

[6] Diagnosing The Permanent Vegetative State by Ronald Cranford, MD

[7] http://content.nejm.org/cgi/content/abstract/330/21/1499

[8] Wade, DT; Johnston, C (1999). "The permanent vegetative state: Practical guidance on diagnosis and management". *BMJ (Clinical research ed.)* **319** (7213): 841–4. doi:10.1136/bmj.319.7213.841. PMC 1116668. PMID 10496834.

[9] *Guidance on diagnosis and management: Report of a working party of the Royal College of Physicians.* Royal College of Physicians: London. 1996.

[10] Bryan Jennett. *The Vegetative State: Medical facts, ethical and legal dilemmas* (PDF). University of Glasgow: Scotland. Retrieved 2007-11-09.

[11] *Post-coma unresponsiveness (Vegetative State): a clinical framework for diagnosis.* National Health and Medical Research Council (NHMRC): Canberra. 2003.

[12] Jennett, B (2002). "Editorial: The vegetative state. The definition, diagnosis, prognosis and pathology of this state are discussed, together with the legal implications". *British Medical Journal* **73** (4): 355–357. doi:10.1136/jnnp.73.4.355. Retrieved 2012-06-11.

[13] Nell Boyce (July 8, 2000). "Is anyone in there?". *New Scientist*: 36.

[14] Schapira, Anthony (December 18, 2006). *Neurology and Clinical Neuroscience.* Mosby. p. 126. ISBN 978-0323033541.

[15] Mirsattari SM, Hammond RR, Sharpe MD, Leung FY, Young GB (April 2004). "Myoclonic status epilepticus following repeated oral ingestion of colloidal silver". *Neurology* **62** (8): 1408–10. doi:10.1212/01.WNL.0000120671.73335.EC. PMID 15111684.

[16] K Andrews, L Murphy, R Munday, and C Littlewood (1996-07-06). "Misdiagnosis of the vegetative state: retrospective study in a rehabilitation unit". *British Medical Journal* **313** (7048): 13–16. doi:10.1136/bmj.313.7048.13. PMC 2351462. PMID 8664760.

[17] Giacino JT, et al. (2002). "Unknown title". *Neurology* **58** (3): 349–353. doi:10.1212/wnl.58.3.349. PMID 11839831.

[18] Owen AM, Coleman MR, Boly M, Davis MH, Laureys S, and Pickard JD (2006-09-08). "Detecting awareness in the vegetative state". *Science* **313** (5792): 1402. doi:10.1126/science.1130197. PMID 16959998.

[19] "Vegetative patient 'communicates': A patient in a vegetative state can communicate just through using her thoughts, according to research". BBC News. September 7, 2006. Retrieved 2008-08-14.

[20] Stein R (September 8, 2006). "Vegetative patient's brain active in test: Unprecedented experiment shows response to instructions to imagine playing tennis". *San Francisco Chronicle.* Retrieved 2007-09-26.

[21] Willful Modulation of Brain Activity in Disorders of Consciousness at nejm.org

[22] Richard Alleyne and Martin Beckford, Patients in 'vegetative' state can think and communicate,*Telegraph* (United Kingdom), Feb 4, 2010

[23] Cruse Damian; et al. "Bedside detection of awareness in the vegetative state: a cohort study". *The Lancet.* doi:10.1016/S0140-6736(11)61224-5.

[24] Dolce, Giuliano; Sazbon, Leon (2002). *The post-traumatic vegetative state.* ISBN 9781588901163.

[25] Georgiopoulos M, et al. (2010). "Vegetative state and minimally conscious state: a review of the therapeutic interventions". *Stereotact Funct Neurosurg* **88** (4): 199–207. doi:10.1159/000314354. PMID 20460949.

[26] Georgiopoulos, M; Katsakiori, P; Kefalopoulou, Z; Ellul, J; Chroni, E; Constantoyannis, C (2010). "Vegetative state and minimally conscious state: a review of the therapeutic interventions.". *Stereotactic and functional neurosurgery* **88** (4): 199–207. doi:10.1159/000314354. PMID 20460949.

[27] Snyman, N; London, K; Howman-Giles, R; Gill, D; Gillis, J; Scheinberg, A; et al. (2010). "Zolpidem for persistent vegetative state--a placebo-controlled trial in pediatrics". *Neuropediatrics* **41** (5): 223–227. doi:10.1055/s-0030-1269893. PMID 21210338.

[28] Whyte, J; Myers, R (2009). "Incidence of clinically significant responses to zolpidem among patients with disorders of consciousness: a preliminary placebo controlled trial". *Am J Phys Med Rehab* **88** (5): 410–418. doi:10.1097/PHM.0b013e3181a0e3a0. PMID 19620954.

[29] Hirsch, Joy (2005-05-02). "Raising consciousness". *The Journal of Clinical Investigation* (American Society for Clinical Investigation) **115** (5): 1102. doi:10.1172/JCI25320. PMC 1087197. PMID 15864333.

[30] Ernst Kretschmer (1940). "Das apallische Syndrom". *Neurol. Psychiat* **169**: 576–579. doi:10.1007/BF02871384.

[31] B Jennett and F Plum (1972). "Persistent vegetative state after brain damage: A syndrome in search of a name". *The Lancet* **1** (7753): 734–737. doi:10.1016/S0140-6736(72)90242-5. PMID 4111204.

[32] Appel on Betancourt v. Trinitas

[33] Richard Alleyne and Martin Beckford, Patients in 'vegetative' state can think and communicate, *Telegraph* (United Kingdom), Feb 4, 2010

[34] "1973 Sexual Assault Victim Aruna Shanbaug passes away in Mumbai". news.biharprabha.com. 18 May 2015. Retrieved 18 May 2015.

• Canavero S, Massa-Micon B, Cauda F, Montanaro E (May 2009). "Bifocal extradural cortical stimulation-induced recovery of consciousness in the permanent post-traumatic vegetative state". *J Neurol* **256** (5): 834–6. doi:10.1007/s00415-009-5019-4.

• Canavero S. Textbook of therapeutic cortical stimulation. New York: Nova Science, 2009

2.16.11   References

This article contains text from the NINDS public domain pages on TBI. and .

• Borthwick C (Fall 1996). "The permanent vegetative state: ethical crux, medical fiction?". *Issues Law Med.* **12** (2): 167–85. The author questions the validity of most PVS diagnoses, and the validity of the basic nosology. The fulltext is available on the author's website.

• Laureys, Steven (2000). "The neural correlate of (un)awareness: lessons from the vegetative state". *Cyclotron Research Center and Department of Neurology* **B30**.

• Matsuda, W.; Matsumura, A.; Komatsu, Y.; Yanaka, K.; Nose, T (2003). "Awakenings from persistent vegetative state: report of three cases with Parkinsonism and brain stem lesions on MRI". *Journal of Neurology, Neurosurgery and Psychiatry* **74** (11): 1571–3. doi:10.1136/jnnp.74.11.1571. PMC 1738238. PMID 14617720.

• Owen, A.M.; Menon, D.K.; Johnsrude, I.S.; Bor, D.; Scott, SK; Manly, T; Williams, EJ; Mummery, C; Pickard, JD (2002). "Detecting residual cognitive function in persistent vegetative state". *Neurocase* **8** (5): 394–403. doi:10.1076/neur.8.4.394.16184. PMID 12499414.

• Boly, M.; Faymonville, ME; Peigneux, P; Lambermont, B; Damas, P; Del Fiore, G; Degueldre, C; Franck, G; et al. (2004). "Auditory Processing in Severely Brain Injured Patients". *Arch Neurol* **61** (2): 233–238. doi:10.1001/archneur.61.2.233. PMID 14967772.

• Emmett, P. A. (1989). "A Biblico-Ethical Response to the Question of Withdrawing Fluid and Nutrition from Individuals in the Persistent Vegetative State" **4–5**. pp. 248–249.

• Ashwal, S.; The Multi-Society Task Force On Pvs (1994). "Medical Aspects of the Persistent Vegetative

State— Second of Two Parts". *N Engl J Med* **330** (22): 1572–1579. doi:10.1056/NEJM199406023302206. PMID 8177248.

• Owen, A.M.; Coleman, M.R.; Johnsrude, I.S.; Menon, D.K.; Rodd, JM; Davis, MH; Taylor, K; Pickard, JD (2005). "Residual auditory function in persistent vegetative state: A combined PET and fMRI study". *Neuropsychological Rehabilitation* **15** (3–4): 290–306. doi:10.1080/09602010443000579. PMID 16350973.

• Laureys, S.; Faymonville, M.E.; Peigneux, P.; Menon, D.K.; Lambermont, B; Del Fiore, G; Degueldre, C; Aerts, J; et al. (2002). "Cortical processing of noxious somatosensory stimuli in the persistent vegetative state". *Neuroimage* **17** (2): 732–741. doi:10.1016/S1053-8119(02)91236-X. PMID 12377148.

• Sarà, M.; Sacco, S.; Cipolla, F.; Onorati, P.; Scoppetta, C; Albertini, G; Carolei, A (2007). "An unexpected recovery from permanent vegetative state". *Brain Injury* **21** (1): 101–103. doi:10.1080/02699050601151761. PMID 17364525.

• Schiff, N.D.; Ribary, U.; Moreno, D.R.; Beattie, B.; Kronberg, E; Blasberg, R; Giacino, J; McCagg, C; et al. (2002). "Residual cerebral activity and behavioural fragments can remain in the persistently vegetative brain". *Brain* **125** (Pt 6): 1210–1234. doi:10.1093/brain/awf131. PMID 12023311.

• "Diagnosis and management: Report of a working party of the Royal College of Physicians". *Royal College of Physicians*. 1996.

• Canavero S, et al. (2009). "Recovery of consciousness following bifocal extradural cortical stimulation in a permanently vegetative patient". *Journal of Neurology* **256** (5): 834–6. doi:10.1007/s00415-009-5019-4. PMID 19252808.

• Canavero S (editor) (2009). *Textbook of therapeutic cortical stimulation*. New York: Nova Science.

2.16.12 Further reading

• Connolly, Kate. Car crash victim trapped in a coma for 23 years was conscious, *The Guardian*, November 23, 2009.

• Hall, Alan. 'I screamed, but there was nothing to hear': Man trapped in 23-year 'coma' reveals horror of being unable to tell doctors he was conscious, *Daily Mail*, November 23, 2009.

• Machado, Calixto, et al A Cuban Perspective on Management of Persistent Vegetative State. *MEDICC Review 2012;14(1):44–48.*

2.17   Pupillary reflex

Pupillary reflex refers to one of the reflexes associated with pupillary function.

Types include:

• Pupillary light reflex

• Accommodation reflex

See also:

• Pupillary response

Although pupillary dilation is not usually called a "reflex", it is still usually considered a part of this topic.

Adjustment to close-range vision is known as "the near response", while inhibition of the ciliary muscle is known as the "far response".

In "the near response" there are three processes that occur to focus an image on the retina. Convergence of the eyes, or the orientation of the visual axis of each eye towards an object in order to focus its image on each fovea, is the first of the three responses. This can be observed by the cross-eyed movement of the eyes when a finger is held up in front of a face and moved towards the face. Next, constriction of the pupil occurs. Because the lens cannot refract light rays at the edges well, the image produced by the lens is blurry around the edges so the pupil constricts when one attempts to focus on nearby objects. Lastly, accommodation of the lens occurs. This is an alteration in the curvature of the lens that allows focus on a nearby object.[1]

2.17.1   References

[1] Saladin, Kenneth S. Anatomy & Physiology: The Unity of Form and Function. 6th ed. New York: McGraw-Hill, 202. 617. Print.

2.18   Unconsciousness

See also: Unconscious mind

Unconsciousness is a state which occurs when the ability to maintain an awareness of self and environment is lost. It involves a complete or near-complete lack of responsiveness to people and other environmental stimuli.[1]

Loss of consciousness should *not* be confused with the notion of the psychoanalytic unconscious or cognitive processes (e.g., implicit cognition) that take place outside of awareness, and with altered states of consciousness, such as delirium (when the person is confused and only partially responsive to the environment), normal sleep, hypnosis, and other altered states in which the person responds to stimuli.

Unconsciousness may occur as the result of traumatic brain injury, brain hypoxia (e.g., due to a brain infarction or cardiac arrest), severe poisoning with drugs that depress the activity of the central nervous system (e.g., alcohol and other hypnotic or sedative drugs), severe fatigue, and other causes.

There is a theory that unconsciousness occurs when different regions of the brain inhibit one another.[2]

2.18.1   Law and medicine

In jurisprudence, unconsciousness may entitle the criminal defendant to the defense of automatism, i.e. a state uncontrollably of one's own actions, an excusing condition that allows a defendant to argue that they should not be held criminally liable for their actions or omissions. In most countries, courts must consider whether unconsciousness in a situation can be accepted as a defense; it can vary from case to case. Hence epileptic seizures, neurological dysfunctions and sleepwalking may be considered acceptable excusing conditions because the loss of control is not foreseeable, but falling asleep (especially while driving or during any other safety-critical activity), may not be because natural sleep rarely overcomes an ordinary person without warning.

In many countries, it is presumed that someone who is less than fully conscious cannot give consent to anything. This can be relevant in cases of sexual behavior, euthanasia or patients giving informed consent with regard to starting or stopping a treatment.

Laws in some countries require that first responders, EMT, or paramedics obtain consent from an injured person who is conscious before they initiate patient care. In most situations where the injured person is deemed unconscious, consent is implied and the emergency service provider is free to provide care.

2.18.2   See also

- Coma

- Do not resuscitate

- Fainting

- Greyout

- Hypnosis

- Living will

- Shallow water blackout

- Sleep

- Somnophilia

- Syncope

- Traumatic brain injury

2.18.3   References

[1] http://www.nlm.nih.gov/cgi/mesh/2009/MB_cgi?field= uid&term=D014474

[2] http://www.bbc.co.uk/news/ science-environment-13751783

2.19   Uniform Determination of Death Act

The **Uniform Determination of Death Act** (**UDDA**) is a model state law that was approved for the United States in 1981 by the National Conference of Commissioners on Uniform State Laws, in cooperation with the American Medical Association, the American Bar Association, and the President's Commission for the Study of Ethical Problems in Medicine and Biomedical and Behavioral Research. The act has since been adopted by most US states and is intended "to provide a comprehensive and medically sound basis for determining death in all situations". Brain death is a different condition that persistent vegetative state. Due to better seat belt use, bicycle helmets, and the general decrease in violent crime, there are lower numbers of brain deaths now than historically. Donation after cardiac death (DCD) is a new protocol applied when there is severe neurologic injury but the patent does not meet the criteria for brain death.

The three sections of the Act proposed for enactment read as follows .:

2.19.1   Section 1

Determination of Death. An individual who has sustained either (1) irreversible cessation of circulatory and respiratory functions, or (2) irreversible cessation of all functions of the entire brain, including the brain stem, is dead. A determination of death must be made in accordance with accepted medical standards.

2.19.2 Section 2

Uniformity of Construction and Application. This Act shall be applied and construed to effectuate its general purpose to make uniform the law with respect to the subject of this Act among states enacting it.

2.19.3 See also

- List of Uniform Acts (United States)

2.19.4 External links

- Maine's Codification of this Act
- Draft of the Act by the NCCUSL
- NCCUSL Home Page
- UDDA explained by HealthCare.Findlaw.com

2.20 Vegetative symptoms

Not to be confused with Vegetative state.

Vegetative symptoms are disturbances of a person's functions necessary to maintain life (vegetative functions). These disturbances are most commonly seen in mood disorders, and are part of the diagnostic criteria for depression, but also appear in other conditions.[1]

Vegetative symptoms in a patient with typical depression include:[2]

- Weight loss and anorexia
- Insomnia
- Fatigue and low energy
- Inattention

2.20.1 Reversed vegetative symptoms

Reversed vegetative symptoms include only oversleeping (*hypersomnia*) and overeating (*hyperphagia*), as compared to insomnia and loss of appetite. These features are characteristic of *atypical depression* (AD).

However, there have been studies[3] claiming that these symptoms alone are sufficient to diagnose the condition of AD.

2.20.2 See also

- Sleep disorder

2.20.3 References

[1] Griffin, JB Jr. (1990). "Chapter 205: Psychological Disturbances of Vegetative Function". In Walker, HK; Hall, WD; Hurst, JW. *Clinical Methods: The History, Physical, and Laboratory Examinations* (3rd ed.) (Boston: Butterworths) http://www.ncbi.nlm.nih.gov/books/NBK318/. Missing or empty |title= (help)

[2] Carey, William. "Physician's Guide to Recognition and Treatment of Depression". *Cleveland Clinic*. Retrieved 4 September 2014. Detection of an MDE in the context of debilitating medical illness is often difficult because the vegetative symptoms of depression (anorexia, insomnia, fatigue, and impaired attention) can occur as manifestations of severe medical or surgical illness itself.

[3] Benazzi F (December 2002). "Can only reversed vegetative symptoms define atypical depression?". *Eur Arch Psychiatry Clin Neurosci* **252** (6): 288–93. doi:10.1007/s00406-002-0395-0. PMID 12563537.

2.21 Vestibulo–ocular reflex

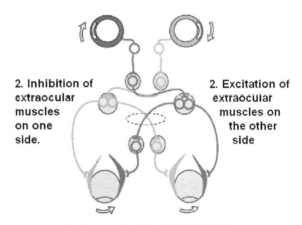

The vestibulo-ocular reflex. A rotation of the head is detected, which triggers an inhibitory signal to the extraocular muscles on one side and an excitatory signal to the muscles on the other side. The result is a compensatory movement of the eyes.

The **vestibulo-ocular reflex** (**VOR**), sometimes known as but not completely synonymous with[1] the **oculocephalic reflex** (which itself is colloquially known as the "doll's head reflex" and is used to assess the health of coma patients, along with VOR)[1] is a reflex eye movement that elicits eye movement by stimulating the vestibular system. This reflex functions to stabilize images on the retinas (in yoked vision) during head movement by producing eye movements in the direction opposite to head movement, thus preserving the image on the center of the visual field(s). For example, when the head moves to the right, the eyes move to the left, and vice versa. Since slight head movement is present all the time, the VOR is very important for stabilizing vision: patients whose VOR is impaired find it difficult to read using print, because they cannot stabilize the eyes during small head tremors, and also because damage to the VOR can cause vestibular nystagmus.[2] The VOR does not depend on visual input. It can be elicited by caloric (hot or cold) stimulation of the inner ear, and works even in total darkness or when the eyes are closed. However, in the presence of light, the fixation reflex is also added to the movement.[3]

In other animals, the gravity organs and eyes are strictly connected. A fish, for instance, moves its eyes by reflex when its tail is moved. Humans have semicircular canals, neck muscle "stretch" receptors, and the utricle (gravity organ). Though the semicircular canals cause most of the reflexes which are responsive to acceleration, the maintaining of balance is mediated by the stretch of neck muscles and the pull of gravity on the utricle (otolith organ) of the inner ear.[3]

The VOR has both rotational and translational aspects. When the head rotates about any axis (horizontal, vertical, or torsional) distant visual images are stabilized by rotating the eyes about the same axis, but in the opposite direction.[4] When the head translates, for example during walking, the visual fixation point is maintained by rotating gaze direction in the opposite direction, by an amount that depends on distance.[5]

2.21.1   Circuit

The VOR is ultimately driven by signals from the vestibular apparatus in the inner ear. The semicircular canals detect head rotation and drive the rotational VOR, whereas the otoliths detect head translation and drive the translational VOR. The main "direct path" neural circuit for the horizontal rotational VOR is fairly simple. It starts in the vestibular system, where semicircular canals get activated by head rotation and send their impulses via the vestibular nerve (cranial nerve VIII) through Scarpa's ganglion and end in the vestibular nuclei in the brainstem. From these nuclei, fibers cross to the contralateral cranial nerve VI nucleus (abducens nucleus). There they synapse with 2 addi-

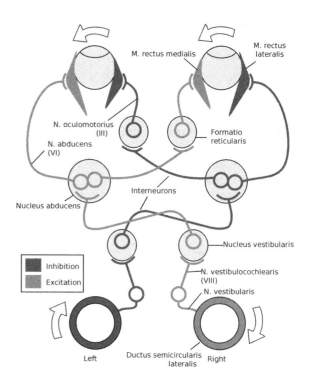

tional pathways. One pathway projects directly to the lateral rectus of eye via the abducens nerve. Another nerve tract projects from the abducens nucleus by the medial longitudinal fasciculus to the contralateral oculomotor nucleus, which contains motorneurons that drive eye muscle activity, specifically activating the medial rectus muscle of the eye through the oculomotor nerve.

Another pathway (not in picture) directly projects from the vestibular nucleus through the ascending tract of Dieters to the ipsilateral medial rectus motoneuron. In addition there are inhibitory vestibular pathways to the ipsilateral abducens nucleus. However no direct vestibular neuron to medial rectus motoneuron pathway exists.[6]

Similar pathways exist for the vertical and torsional components of the VOR.

In addition to these direct pathways, which drive the velocity of eye rotation, there is an indirect pathway that builds up the position signal needed to prevent the eye from rolling back to center when the head stops moving. This pathway is particularly important when the head is moving slowly, because here position signals dominate over velocity signals. David A. Robinson discovered that the eye muscles require this dual velocity-position drive, and also proposed that it must arise in the brain by mathematically integrating the velocity signal and then sending the resulting position signal to the motoneurons. Robinson was correct: the 'neural integrator' for horizontal eye position was found in the nucleus prepositus hypoglossi[7] in the medulla, and the neural integrator for vertical and torsional eye positions was found in the interstitial nucleus of Cajal[8] in the midbrain. The same neural integrators also generate eye position for other conjugate eye movements such as saccades and smooth pursuit.

Excitatory example

For instance, if the head is turned clockwise as seen from above, then excitatory impulses are sent from the semicircular canal on the right side via the vestibular nerve (cranial nerve VIII) through Scarpa's ganglion and end in the right vestibular nuclei in the brainstem. From this nuclei excitatory fibers cross to the left abducens nucleus. There they project and stimulate the lateral rectus of the left eye via the abducens nerve. In addition, by the medial longitudinal fasciculus and oculomotor nuclei, they activate the medial rectus muscles on the right eye. As a result, both eyes will turn counterclockwise.

Furthermore, some neurons from the right vestibular nucleus directly stimulate the right medial rectus motoneurons, and inhibits the right abducens nucleus.

2.21.2 Speed

The vestibulo-ocular reflex needs to be fast: for clear vision, head movement must be compensated almost immediately; otherwise, vision corresponds to a photograph taken with a shaky hand. To achieve clear vision, signals from the semicircular canals are sent as directly as possible to the eye muscles: the connection involves only three neurons, and is correspondingly called the *three neuron arc*. Using these direct connections, eye movements lag the head movements by less than 10 ms,[9] and thus the vestibulo-ocular reflex is one of the fastest reflexes in the human body.

2.21.3 Gain

The "gain" of the VOR is defined as the change in the eye angle divided by the change in the head angle during the head turn. Ideally the gain of the rotational VOR is 1.0. The gain of the horizontal and vertical VOR is usually close to 1.0, but the gain of the torsional VOR (rotation around the line of sight) is generally low.[4] The gain of the translational VOR has to be adjusted for distance, because of the geometry of motion parallax. When the head translates, the angular direction of near targets changes faster than the angular direction of far targets.[5]

If the gain of the VOR is wrong (different from 1)—for example, if eye muscles are weak, or if a person puts on

a new pair of eyeglasses—then head movement results in image motion on the retina, resulting in blurred vision. Under such conditions, motor learning adjusts the gain of the VOR to produce more accurate eye motion. This is what is referred to as VOR adaptation.

Ethanol consumption can disrupt the VOR, reducing dynamic visual acuity.[10]

2.21.4 Testing

This reflex can be tested by the *Rapid head impulse test* or *Halmagyi-Curthoys-test*, in which the head is rapidly moved to the side with force, and is controlled if the eyes succeed to remain looking in the same direction. When the function of the right balance system is reduced, by a disease or by an accident, quick head movement to the right cannot be sensed properly anymore. As a consequence, no compensatory eye movement is generated, and the patient cannot fixate a point in space during this rapid head movement.

Another way of testing the VOR response is a caloric reflex test, which is an attempt to induce nystagmus (compensatory eye movement in the absence of head motion) by pouring cold or warm water into the ear. Also available is bi-thermal air caloric irrigations, in which warm and cool air is administered into the ear.

Comatose patients

In comatose patients, once it has been determined that the cervical spine is intact, a test of the vestibulo-ocular reflex can be performed by turning the head to one side. If the brainstem is intact, the eyes will move conjugately away from the direction of turning (as if still looking at the examiner rather than fixed straight ahead). Negative "doll's eyes" would stay fixed midorbit, and having negative "doll's eyes" is therefore a sign that a comatose patient's brainstem is functionally not intact.

Testing complications

Currently, vestibulo-ocular reflexes can only be comprehensively tested in specially equipped laboratories. The tests sometimes provide valuable diagnostic information; however, the tests can be time-consuming and expensive to administer. The scleral search coil can be used to assess the vestibulo-ocular reflex.

2.21.5 Role of cerebellum

The cerebellum is essential for motor learning to correct the VOR in order to ensure accurate eye movement. Motor learning in the VOR is in many ways analogous to classical eyeblink conditioning, since the circuits are homologous and the molecular mechanisms are similar.

2.21.6 See also

- Caloric reflex test
- Image stabilization
- Pursuit movement
- Semicircular canals
- Vestibular system
- Vestibulocerebellar syndrome

2.21.7 References

[1] http://www.ncbi.nlm.nih.gov/pmc/articles/PMC1031870/pdf/jnnpsyc00551-0015.pdf

[2] http://www.dizziness-and-balance.com/practice/nystagmus/vestibular.html

[3] "Sensory Reception: Human Vision: Structure and function of the Human Eye" vol. 27, p. 179 Encyclopaedia Britannica, 1987

[4] Crawford, JD; Vilis, T (Mar 1991). "Axes of eye rotation and Listing's law during rotations of the head.". *Journal of neurophysiology* **65** (3): 407–23. PMID 2051188.

[5] Angelaki, DE (Jul 2004). "Eyes on target: what neurons must do for the vestibuloocular reflex during linear motion.". *Journal of neurophysiology* **92** (1): 20–35. doi:10.1152/jn.00047.2004. PMID 15212435.

[6] Straka H, Dieringer N (2004). "Basic organization principles of the VOR: lessons from frogs". *Prog. Neurobiol.* **73** (4): 259–309. doi:10.1016/j.pneurobio.2004.05.003. PMID 15261395.

[7] Cannon, SC; Robinson, DA (May 1987). "Loss of the neural integrator of the oculomotor system from brain stem lesions in monkey.". *Journal of neurophysiology* **57** (5): 1383–409. PMID 3585473.

[8] Crawford, JD; Cadera, W; Vilis, T (Jun 14, 1991). "Generation of torsional and vertical eye position signals by the interstitial nucleus of Cajal.". *Science* **252** (5012): 1551–3. doi:10.1126/science.2047862. PMID 2047862.

[9] Aw, ST; Halmagyi, GM; Haslwanter, T; Curthoys, IS; Yavor, RA; Todd, MJ (Dec 1996). "Three-dimensional vector analysis of the human vestibuloocular reflex in response to high-acceleration head rotations. II. responses in subjects with unilateral vestibular loss and selective semicircular canal occlusion.". *Journal of neurophysiology* **76** (6): 4021–30. PMID 8985897.

[10] Schmäl, F; Thiede, O; Stoll, W (Sep 2003). "Effect of ethanol on visual-vestibular interactions during vertical linear body acceleration.". *Alcoholism, clinical and experimental research* **27** (9): 1520–6. doi:10.1097/01.ALC.0000087085.98504.8C. PMID 14506414.

2.21.8 External links

- (Video) Head Impulse Testing site (vHIT) Site with thorough information about vHIT
- Motor Learning in the VOR in Mice at edboyden.org
- Review on VOR adaptation via slides at Johns Hopkins University
- Vestibulo-Ocular Reflex at the US National Library of Medicine Medical Subject Headings (MeSH)
- Center for Integration of Medicine and Innovative Technology - Testing device development
- *ent/482* at eMedicine - "Vestibuloocular Reflex Testing"
- Depiction of Oculocephalic and Caloric reflexes
-
-

Chapter 3

Text and image sources, contributors, and licenses

3.1 Text

- **Brain death** *Source:* https://en.wikipedia.org/wiki/Brain_death?oldid=688315905 *Contributors:* The Anome, Youssefsan, Roadrunner, Someone else, Patrick, Karada, NuclearWinner, Ams80, Ahoerstemeier, Ronz, Julesd, Kaihsu, Emperorbma, WhisperToMe, Wik, Pakaran, Slawojarek, Robbot, Ktotam, Ojigiri~enwiki, Blainster, Benc, Diberri, Connelly, Ksheka, Reub2000, Spencer195, Jfdwolff, Jrdioko, Fuzzy Logic, Abu badali, HorsePunchKid, Gunnar Larsson, Bk0, Mariko~enwiki, Hydrox, Rupertslander, Smyth, El C, JRM, Kormoran, Arcadian, Qazzx, MPerel, ADM, AnnaP, Andrewpmk, Osmodiar, ReyBrujo, Garzo, Macgruder, PullUpYourSocks, Hondje~enwiki, Jeffrey O. Gustafson, Mr Tan, Benbest, Kelisi, Mangojuice, Mandarax, Graham87, NixonB, BD2412, Stevenplunkett, Dwaipayanc, Sjö, Rjwilmsi, JoshuacUK, FlaBot, Jeepo~enwiki, Mister Matt, JdforresterBot, Chobot, DVdm, YurikBot, HG1, RussBot, Polacrilex, Eleassar, Mccready, Nephron, AGToth, Bibliomaniac15, Sacxpert, SmackBot, McGeddon, Captainahab92, Skizzik, Bluebot, John Reaves, Yidisheryid, Clicketyclack, Mksword, KL-Lvr283, Tktktk, Akish~enwiki, Stupid Corn, Jack O'Neill, Kiwi8, Gunstar hero, Blackhawk charlie2003, Snorkelman, Ale jrb, JohnCD, Ruslik0, Green caterpillar, Alton, Michaelas10, DumbBOT, AntiVandalBot, Salgueiro~enwiki, Qwerty Binary, Magioladitis, Bongwarrior, JamesBWatson, Animum, EagleFan, Drslaw, JaGa, WLU, Yobol, Mmoneypenny, Skepticus, El0i, Bongomatic, Ijustam, Mikael Häggström, Mohrflies, Yaoi Kat na-no-da, Vranak, AlnoktaBOT, Philip Trueman, TXiKiBoT, Anonymous Dissident, Nazgul02, Wasted Sapience, Riversong, Doc James, YURiN, Qraali, SieBot, Demong, Briefer, Skylark42, Jrastronomer, Flyer22 Reborn, MaynardClark, Mailman9, Sean.hoyland, Soulrefrain, ClueBot, Samkir, Mechatronik, DWEvansMD, Osomite, Bde1982, DatRoot, SchreiberBike, Cowardly Lion, JKeck, Dtpeck, Thehotshotpilot, HexaChord, Addbot, DOI bot, Ronhjones, Movingboxes, Ironholds, MrOllie, Proxima Centauri, Quercus solaris, Splodgeness, Tassedethe, Numbo3-bot, Jarble, Luckas-bot, Yobot, Amirobot, DiverDave, AnomieBOT, Funcrunch, Citation bot, Ddstuhlman, Gap9551, Srich32977, Shmona, Onlyafaceinthecrowd, Wiltingfoster, FrescoBot, Zachalope, StaticVision, Rkomorn, Atlantia, Razorbelle, RedBot, Cullen328, Pristino, Suffusion of Yellow, Mean as custard, VernoWhitney, EmausBot, -- -- --, TheGeomaster, Kiwi128, MagicalThinking, Kaiserm, Wingman4l7, Anglais1, Ready, Hummelsang, Senator2029, ClueBot NG, Peter James, SuperCoder, MEDRS, Helpful Pixie Bot, Theoldsparkle, BG19bot, Cranmills, Bcary, Bonkers The Clown, BattyBot, Art348, SamuelRowe, Blex areton, Dexbot, Martinillo, Everything Is Numbers, Morten13ok, Benjips, Isaacsaccount, PraetorianFury, Jag512, Edwardleonardy, Banimelhim, SuperSwaggieSwagger, Abutplead, EtymAesthete, Jaxbax7, Monkbot, Ca2james, BoboMeowCat, Oiyarbepsy, Poiuytrewqvtaatv123321, JasonRobertYoungMD, KasparBot, DenisLedent, Ramirezmony5, Jhgf9876 and Anonymous: 185

- **Disorders of consciousness** *Source:* https://en.wikipedia.org/wiki/Disorders_of_consciousness?oldid=672912537 *Contributors:* Deb, Wouterstomp, Rjwilmsi, SmackBot, WhatamIdoing, Olegwiki, Maralia, Editor2020, Addbot, Citation bot, 1@Di, Razorbelle, Trappist the monk, Whoop whoop pull up, Neøn, MrBill3, IjonTichyIjonTichy, Lewellenks, JRicker,PhD and Anonymous: 8

- **Brain stem death** *Source:* https://en.wikipedia.org/wiki/Brain_stem_death?oldid=680047754 *Contributors:* The Anome, Julesd, FT2, ArnoldReinhold, Cje~enwiki, SteinbDJ, Pol098, Oldelpaso, Graham87, BD2412, PhatRita, Chobot, Hatch68, Bgwhite, JarrahTree, RussBot, Retired username, Lpm, SmackBot, CSZero, Keegan, Radagast83, Lambiam, KX36, Hervegirod, Anupam, Widefox, Catslash, Fabrictramp, R'n'B, Adavidb, Katharineamy, CardinalDan, Wikiisawesome, DavidWEvans, Greswik, Naravorgaara, Briefer, Skylark42, BNogrady, Brinlong, FunkyDuffy, DWEvansMD, Purplewowies, SchreiberBike, RichardWild, UnCatBot, Tcncv, Tharyps the Molossian, Mhadj001, Chzz, Bwrs, Teles, Yobot, KamikazeBot, DiverDave, AnomieBOT, Xqbot, Srich32977, Alamelhuda, Manjel, Hexafluoride, FoxBot, North8000, VernoWhitney, Fiftytwo thirty, GoingBatty, Senator2029, Molestash, VEBott, Widr, Helpful Pixie Bot, Iankp, Lakanal, Morganson691, Sudhamshu50, Iztwoz, JessRadford and Anonymous: 25

- **Caloric reflex test** *Source:* https://en.wikipedia.org/wiki/Caloric_reflex_test?oldid=659862336 *Contributors:* The Anome, Diberri, Chuckster0, HorsePunchKid, Arcadian, Nephron, RDBrown, Pwjb, Jkokavec, Alaibot, WhatamIdoing, Oren0, Nono64, CFCF, Davwillev, Maralia, Wdustbuster, Versus22, Daliemans, Mara Determan, DOI bot, Lightbot, Yobot, Tohd8BohaithuGh1, Citation bot, J04n, Opiance, Citation bot 1, MSymer, Gsarwa, Rocketrod1960, Helpful Pixie Bot, NLMOCPL, Comp.arch, Monkbot and Anonymous: 30

- **Clinical death** *Source:* https://en.wikipedia.org/wiki/Clinical_death?oldid=685910865 *Contributors:* The Anome, Roadrunner, Ixfd64, Karada, Ellywa, Emperorbma, Robbot, Hadal, Jfdwolff, Yekrats, Erich gasboy, Rich Farmbrough, Cohesion, Minority Report, Osmodiar, Gene Nygaard, Greentryst, Benbest, Patman, Graham87, Rjwilmsi, Mister Matt, Margosbot~enwiki, Oggy, Peter Grey, YurikBot, Bullzeye, Irishguy,

Zephalis, Richardcavell, PTSE, Danny-w, Mais oui!, Sacxpert, SmackBot, Amcbride, Imz, Cryobiologist, Dlodge, RDBrown, WikiPedant, Tsca.bot, Kuru, Spencer233416, Andyroo316, Aeternus, Ruslik0, Michaelas10, Anthonyhcole, WikiPrez, Thijs!bot, Krilnon, Cphillipsxyz, Diablod666, GirlForLife, Wiki Raja, RockMFR, Stephanwehner, Ferahgo the Assassin, AlnoktaBOT, Skeptic06, SieBot, StAnselm, Ttony21, Briefer, Rimas Letap, Dlrohrer2003, VQuakr, Deineka, Addbot, Aceofhearts1968, DOI bot, Theleftorium, Diptanshu.D, F Notebook, Tide rolls, Lightbot, OlEnglish, Enjoydrawn, AmeliorationBot, AnomieBOT, Citation bot, Obersachsebot, Srich32977, Citation bot 1, Jonesey95, Jauhienij, DixonDBot, RjwilmsiBot, ZxxZxxZ, H3llBot, Peter M. Brown, Neoprometheus, MusikAnimal, MrBill3, PMorrisUK, Jimw338, Khazar2, TwoTwoHello, 93, Anrnusna, Linuxjava, Monkbot, Ca2james, Oiyarbepsy and Anonymous: 55

- **Coma** *Source:* https://en.wikipedia.org/wiki/Coma?oldid=688343613 *Contributors:* Vicki Rosenzweig, Bryan Derksen, The Anome, Tarquin, RoseParks, ErdemTuzun, Ed Poor, Youssefsan, Rmhermen, Christian List, Zippy, ChrisSteinbach, JohnOwens, Michael Hardy, Booyabazooka, Kwertii, Ixfd64, Karada, Skysmith, Paul A, NuclearWinner, Looxix~enwiki, Ahoerstemeier, Julesd, Kricke, Evercat, Stew2050, Conti, Magnus Bäck, Timwi, Glimz~enwiki, WhisperToMe, Wilianz, David Shay, Head, Betterworld, JonathanDP81, Robbot, Vardion, Samrolken, Danhuby, Texture, Victor, Trevor Johns, GarnetRChaney, Giftlite, DocWatson42, Curps, Jfdwolff, OldakQuill, Erich gasboy, Utcursch, Pgan002, Onco p53, Gscshoyru, Mrdectol, Maikel, Lacrimosus, Discospinster, Rich Farmbrough, FT2, Tristan Schmelcher, Warpflyght, LindsayH, Pavel Vozenilek, Martpol, Diogenes~enwiki, Slokunshialgo, Aecis, Ben Webber, El C, Shanes, Art LaPella, TomStar81, Archfalhwyl, Kormoran, Arcadian, Nk, Holdek, MPerel, Pearle, APPER, Eric Kvaalen, Wouterstomp, Walkerma, RPH, Harej, RainbowOfLight, Metju~enwiki, Richard Weil, Japanese Searobin, Zntrip, Feezo, Dr Gangrene, Firsfron, Roger6106, Peter Beard, WadeSimMiser, Linusthefish, Chochopk, Kelisi, Tslocum, Graham87, BD2412, FreplySpang, Tizio, NekoFever, Vary, Linuxbeak, FlaBot, McAusten, AJR, Gurch, Intgr, ViriiK, Bgwhite, YurikBot, Whoisjohngalt, Gaius Cornelius, Grafen, Welsh, Kvn8907, Mccready, Veimano, Mysid, Ccgrimm, Sooperhotshiz, Encephalon, Rb82, BorgQueen, AGToth, Katieh5584, Sethie, Andrew73, AndrewWTaylor, Dreamstalker, SmackBot, Unschool, Originalbigj, Chazz88, Bomac, Delldot, HalfShadow, Gilliam, Squiddy, Bluebot, ElTchanggo, MalafayaBot, WildCowboy, Scwlong, Amazon10x, TedE, Astroview120mm, Kalathalan, SanderB, SashatoBot, ArglebargleIV, Ex nihil, Optakeover, Doczilla, Manifestation, DabMachine, IvanLanin, Hydra Rider, CapitalR, Drndmc, Fork me, Avapoet, Denstat, Doctormatt, Gogo Dodo, Konstantin3307, Chasingsol, Tawkerbot4, Vanished User jdksfajlasd, Thijs!bot, Epbr123, Malusdei, Mojo Hand, WillMak050389, WastBarktender100, Electron9, Ufwuct, DaveJ7, Nick Number, Borneh, Escarbot, AntiVandalBot, Sun Tzu Eraserhead, Varlet16, Seaphoto, Gary cumberland, StringRay, Quihn, Camptown, BeefRendang, Res2216firestar, Fshafique, JAnDbot, Leuko, PhilKnight, Acroterion, Magioladitis, Bongwarrior, VoABot II, Gfarlow, Catgut, EagleFan, Hveziris, WLU, Ztobor, BP322, Scottalter, Yobol, MartinBot, Helenf, Keith D, Verdatum, Tgeairn, Maurice Carbonaro, Fastspinecho, Igno2, H8jd5, DarkFalls, Anappart, Juliancolton, STBotD, Evb-wiki, S.riccardelli, Treisijs, Xerosoft, Idioma-bot, Migospia, VolkovBot, Macedonian, Autie62, Seattle Skier, Philip Trueman, TXiKiBoT, Mercurywoodrose, Dialh, Valencerian, DennyColt, Leafyplant, Joseph A. Spadaro, LyraCat, Doc James, AlleborgoBot, Kehrbykid, Demarah, Jlsnacks, SieBot, Tbo 157, Rob.bastholm, Flyer22 Reborn, Komusou, Oxymoron83, Hobartimus, DivineBurner, Trip45, Emptymountains, Ryancormack, Dr Joshua Hunt, Beijing Institute, Reaper85, ClueBot, GorillaWarfare, The Thing That Should Not Be, Techdawg667, EoGuy, Meekywiki, Rosuav, Blanchardb, Auntof6, Aua, DragonBot, Jammy0002, Eeekster, 7&6=thirteen, Zeldafreakx86, SchreiberBike, Lindberg, Aitias, Versus22, SoxBot III, DumZiBoT, Simple implication, Helixweb, XLinkBot, Jovianeye, Nepenthes, SilvonenBot, NellieBly, Frood, EEng, Thatguyflint, Addbot, STARTCH, Friginator, Moosehadley, Vishnava, Diptanshu.D, MrOllie, Download, LaaknorBot, Tassedethe, Numbo3-bot, Lightbot, Ben Ben, Legobot, Luckas-bot, ZX81, Yobot, Ptbotgourou, SwisterTwister, Dmarquard, AnomieBOT, DemocraticLuntz, Marauder40, JackieBot, Materialscientist, Citation bot, .غ.دمح24, Panmarko, Obersachsebot, Xqbot, Caseyonfire, Timir2, 4I7.4I7, Sabisue, Humicroav, Mặt trời đỏ, Srich32977, PimRijkee, Call me Bubba, RibotBOT, Sabrebd, Gordonrox24, FrescoBot, Tbarrett027, JMS Old Al, Breadblade, PeterEastern, Citation bot 1, Aldy, Pinethicket, Razorbelle, Biblequiz, Supreme Deliciousness, Bgpaulus, Jauhienij, Mystic.ejoy27, Trappist the monk, Kalaiarasy, HoworHow, Sgt. R.K. Blue, Froestl, Ballet99~enwiki, Mr. High school student, Dharokowns, DARTH SIDIOUS 2, CoffeeLoveGuy, Onel5969, RjwilmsiBot, Fäkalienmartin, EmausBot, John of Reading, Skysmurf, WikitanvirBot, RenamedUser01302013, DavidMCEddy, Rhoruff, Lawl95, Lji1942, Brandmeister, Donner60, Glarkin53, Nebuliser, Kevin.strong, Peter Karlsen, ClueBot NG, JessicaElizabeth, Dr. Persi, LogX, This lousy T-shirt, Vacation9, ShellyBella, Widr, WikiPuppies, Lionhead99, Luke.oscar, Rhydic, BG19bot, Сол-раз, Hz.tiang, Davidiad, MrBill3, Largefoot, Minsbot, Mikeblahblah, Koopatrev, Lucyt345, Dexbot, King jakob c, 93, Geniers, Waeja230, Epicgenius, Joelsimms, GoTzSkIlLz, Siridean, Thusitbegins, Monkbot, Thebigmarn69, Scarlettail, Jhx4mp, Reallypo9, Youniszainal, Mathewhomberger, Gamingforfun365, Alneet, Mike a nike4484, Smartadenya, Adambroseph1 and Anonymous: 455

- **Corneal reflex** *Source:* https://en.wikipedia.org/wiki/Corneal_reflex?oldid=657180711 *Contributors:* Northgrove, Robbot, Bethenco, Christian.B, Arcadian, Oldman~enwiki, Uncle G, TeaDrinker, JarrahTree, Mikepascoe, SmackBot, Jwestbrook, Pwjb, Mat8989, JWaters, Savonnn, Chmee2, Thijs!bot, Kauczuk, STBot, Nono64, J.delanoy, Andreas Carter, Rashka00, Unused0026, SF007, Addbot, Nuvitauy07, Fluffernutter, Tempodivalse, AnomieBOT, Jrobinjapan, Materialscientist, Shirik, Alexchen4836, Inferior Olive, Thecheesykid, ZéroBot, ClueBot NG, Snotbot, Knowledgeforever2, Rytyho usa, Whatarube, Ultimate cosmic evil and Anonymous: 35

- **Do not resuscitate** *Source:* https://en.wikipedia.org/wiki/Do_not_resuscitate?oldid=683781277 *Contributors:* Vicki Rosenzweig, Roadrunner, Patrick, Michael Hardy, MartinHarper, Menchi, Tregoweth, Hike395, DJ Clayworth, Furrykef, Benc, Diberri, Alan Liefting, Nunh-huh, Jfdwolff, Hugh2414, Pascal666, Hob, Erich gasboy, DanielCD, Discospinster, Guanabot, Tronno, Daf, Gregmcpherson, Echuck215, Runtime, BDD, 2004-12-29T22:45Z, Mindmatrix, Pol098, Rjwilmsi, ENeville, Kenkoo1987, 222fjb, Richardcavell, SmackBot, Imz, Prodego, Leki, Kintetsubuffalo, Jellytussle, Bluebot, Persian Poet Gal, Basalisk, Redheaded dude, DocJohnny, W Ed, Minaker, Vanished user 9i39j3, Filippowiki, Ckatz, Joseph Solis in Australia, Gnusmas, President David Palmer, Porterhse, Gregbard, Dadofsam, JamesAM, Epbr123, Bigwyrm, Pcbene, Big Bird, Cattona, AntiVandalBot, Caledones, MastCell, MHarrison, Mofs, Yobol, It Is Me Here, CoJaBo, Bader isu, Kacser, Billinghurst, Doc James, Rob.bastholm, Dawn Bard, Vanished user 82345ijgeke4tg, WRK, Kotabatubara, Jsfouche, Redmarkviolinist, Naima.fatimi, SpoticusKC, Quoth nevermore~enwiki, Binksternet, Trivialist, Coralmizu, Gassy999, Suxamethonium, Proofer47, Thingg, Versus22, DumZiBoT, Life of Riley, Eik Corell, TaalVerbeteraar, Stickee, Good Olfactory, JPINFV, Chzz, Ayman Qasrawi, Legobot, MisterFine, AnomieBOT, Kingpin13, Materialscientist, Quebec99, LilHelpa, CXCV, Meewam, Srich32977, Haltendehand, Tomballguy, Maria Sieglinda von Nudeldorf, Basket of Puppies, Stiepan Pietrov, BloodGrapefruit2, Jaxboy32, Redondomax, Pinethicket, Tinton5, Koc61, RjwilmsiBot, Legalskeptic, Wikipelli, JBOURNE, R.M.McKernan, Jesanj, Hudson Stern, FeatherPluma, ClueBot NG, Легат Ская, Syleth, ElectMayor, Helpful Pixie Bot, TennTwister, Regulov, Dsduggan, MrBill3, Johnny locks sudbury, EricEnfermero, BattyBot, Tutelary, Andycare, Cyberbot II, ChrisGualtieri, Khazar2, Cerabot~enwiki, Casta947, YiFeiBot, Brittly, Cook8530, Carol Eblen, Monkbot, Uշnun Sı ı, Wilsondoug, SXUComm24, Isaacvargas1024098 and Anonymous: 91

- **Electroencephalography** *Source:* https://en.wikipedia.org/wiki/Electroencephalography?oldid=688983919 *Contributors:* Fnielsen, Codeczero,

Jtoomim, Heron, Rsabbatini, Llywrch, Bewildebeast, AFLastra~enwiki, DopefishJustin, Kku, TakuyaMurata, Karada, Ellywa, Ronz, JWSchmidt, BenKovitz, Hgamboa, Omegatron, Topbanana, Shantavira, Kizor, Rolando, Goethean, Pingveno, Ashdurbat, Clngre, Rhombus, Jondel, Geenah, Radomil, Wikibot, Giftlite, DocWatson42, Jfdwolff, Ding~enwiki, Eequor, Dfrankow, Andycjp, Sonjaaa, Beland, Glogger, Simoneau, Bk0, Sayeth, Geenah71, Indolering, Asbestos, Pjacobi, Rama, Kndiaye, Gronky, Bender235, Jaberwocky6669, JustinWick, CanisRufus, RoyBoy, Muntfish, 2005, Army1987, Njyoder, Arcadian, Giraffedata, Forteanajones, Jumbuck, Jcsutton, Arthena, Sjschen, Riana, Hu, Caesura, Snowolf, Cburnett, Vuo, Ceyockey, Bobrayner, OwenX, Barrylb, Rvanschaik, Janbrogger, Robert K S, D.Right, MarcoTolo, Miroku Sanna, Rjwilmsi, Nightscream, Heah, DoctorDog, Lyo, JuneD, EBlack, Brighterorange, FlaBot, Psydoc~enwiki, Intgr, Shooravi~enwiki, A.Warner, Chobot, Celebere, Vyroglyph, YurikBot, Wavelength, Sceptre, Chris Capoccia, Piet Delport, Monito, CanadianCaesar, Eleassar, Rsrikanth05, NawlinWiki, A314268, MrSandman, Deodar~enwiki, Banes, Daniel Mietchen, Balizarde, Supten, Wknight94, Rwxrwxrwx, D'Agosta, Esprit15d, Colin, Back ache, Dontaskme, AGToth, Axfangli, Eykanal, Macdorman, SmackBot, PSYBIRD1, Gilliam, Mikage31582, Sonicandfffan, Teemu08, Kxra, Tekhnofiend, Zsinj, Can't sleep, clown will eat me, Милан Јелисавчић, Lansey, Jumping cheese, Jdlambert, Hoof Hearted, Kieranfox, Xieliwei, Spiritia, SashatoBot, Zeraeph, Gleng, JorisvS, SandyGeorgia, Th1alb, DabMachine, Chephyr, Iridescent, Michaelbusch, Hewn, AVJP619, Chirality, AbsolutDan, Wikifarzin, Mellery, XApple, CmdrObot, Ilphin, CBM, WeggeBot, Jefchip, Cydebot, Kanags, Anthonyhcole, Beefnut, Dancter, Deele, Kozuch, Thijs!bot, Epbr123, Headbomb, JustAGal, CharlotteWebb, Mmortal03, Escarbot, Ismailmohammed, KrakatoaKatie, Simbven, MER-C, SiobhanHansa, VoABot II, Arno Matthias, Tonyfaull, Fabrictramp, Thuglas, Alex Spade, LookingGlass, Middleman 77, Thibbs, Vssun, DerHexer, Hbent, Ashishbhatnagar72, Mmoneypenny, CliffC, BetBot~enwiki, Jim.henderson, Nikpapag, CommonsDelinker, Gyro2222, PCock, Trusilver, Adavidb, Peter Chastain, Hans Dunkelberg, Tikiwont, Maurice Carbonaro, Mike.lifeguard, Extransit, Kpmiyapuram, Mrs.meganmmc, LordAnubisBOT, Longouyang, Notreallydavid, Mikael Häggström, Plasticup, LittleHow, Timokeefe, STBotD, DorganBot, Xetrov, Davecrosby uk, Poorman1, Mlewis000, LLcopp, VolkovBot, Mbmaciver, Jones2, TXiKiBoT, Malinaccier, Kww, LabFox, Rei-bot, Ask123, Lradrama, Imasleepviking, Zeuszeus1122, KUutela, Mirasoledrecovery, Synthebot, Lova Falk, Temporaluser, Doc James, Simbamford, Jasontable, Nabinkm, SieBot, Fchapotot, Meightysix, Keilana, Berserkerus, Shwmtpf, Rena Silverman, OKBot, Correogsk, Savie Kumara, Michael Tangermann, Emptymountains, Tatterfly, ImageRemovalBot, Twinsday, Martarius, Elassint, ClueBot, Marleneklingeman, Fyyer, The Thing That Should Not Be, Journals88, Mild Bill Hiccup, Callumny, Goldkingtut5, Aorwing, Jumbolino, EeepEeep, Ryan.rakib, Keysanger, Lartoven, Sun Creator, M.O.X, Kaiba, ChrisHamburg, Roberrific, Sribulusu, Delldot on a public computer, Theo177, Elenaschifirnet, XLinkBot, Staticshakedown, EastTN, Rror, Legija, Facts707, Redhorseby, Addbot, DOI bot, Zefryl, Jncraton, Fieldday-sunday, Ethanpet113, Leszek Jańczuk, Diptanshu.D, Dranorter, Looie496, MrOllie, Redheylin, Debresser, Quercus solaris, TangLab, Urness.sam, Numbo3-bot, Katharine908, Lightbot, Wojder, Filip em, Luckas-bot, Yobot, II MusLiM HyBRiD II, Sineenuchn, AnomieBOT, Tryptofish, Ciphers, Rjanag, Jim1138, Bluerasberry, Materialscientist, RobertEves92, Citation bot, Adnan niazi, Zad68, Capricorn42, Cambyzez nl~enwiki, Loveless, The Evil IP address, GrouchoBot, Taylorchas, RibotBOT, Stratocracy, Btait101, Uhhhhhno, Sirmikey, FrescoBot, Tobby72, Odissea, Dger, Steve Quinn, Endoran, Darrellx, Citation bot 1, Citation bot 4, Scidata, Dimo400, ImageTagBot, Veronica Roberts, BrandonSargent, Σ, TjeerdB, Corinne68, TobeBot, Trappist the monk, Datahaki, Namita123, Paiamshadi, Cronides2, Cp72, Solzhenitsyn1, RjwilmsiBot, Afowle, EmausBot, Kfederme, John of Reading, Yanglifu90, GoingBatty, Zagoury, TuHan-Bot, Robertmabell, Scrane72, Ylwarrior, Schulze-bonhage, Midas02, Whet Under The Ears, Rcsprinter123, Δ, Srujan1001, Whelanrobwiki, Neuro11, Alonker, Geoffrey-May, ClueBot NG, Horoporo, Colapeninsula, Beyondsquirrelly, Ariangiovanni, Jj1236, Cntras, Save me, Barry!, FiachraByrne, Alphalobe, Widr, Helpful Pixie Bot, XXLOLDAXx, Titodutta, Bibcode Bot, LizzardKitty, BG19bot, Virtualerian, MerryMilkMan, Bruce4949, Neøn, F Woodruff, Rstdenis, Exercisephys, KPFrerking, Glacialfox, Fernandopestana, Welpeo, Enirpmet, Darkcharmr, BrightStarSky, Dexbot, Hmainsbot1, Mogism, Needcnest, CuriousMind01, TwoTwoHello, 93, Matt-in-a-hat-42, Mark viking, River2012wiki, Scareccrow, Etch6, Mzoltan24, XABXCO, Evano1van, Dkz999, Morozless, Dalli 2013, Omphalosskeptic, I3roly, Rhythm1140, Monkbot, BirthOfJesus, Lara comb, Jaun-Jimenez, Clathrin, Globalglobes, Minuit2400, Poiuytrewqvtaatv123321, Dr.Ashlesh.P, BESA GmbH, Andre at besa, WhyPrivate?, Me.agmohit, Dfleur, Quinto Simmaco, KasparBot, VaibhavGandhi1, Ashfaquememon, Milly shepp, Wolk777, Haodong123, Blacknick and Anonymous: 415

- **Information-theoretic death** *Source:* https://en.wikipedia.org/wiki/Information-theoretic_death?oldid=678219593 *Contributors:* Ciphergoth, Evercat, Charles Matthews, David Gerard, Everyking, Brianhe, Localhost00, Stuartyeates, Simetrical, Mindmatrix, Benbest, Qwertyus, That Guy, From That Show!, SmackBot, Cryobiologist, Bluebot, Sbharris, Bigturtle, Drphilharmonic, Petr Kopač, Rabidchipmunk666, Myncknm, Dkowalski, Tkgd2007, Pwnage8, Flyer22 Reborn, Tesi1700, RMerkle, Addbot, Tornsubject, Bwrs, Jarble, Yobot, AnomieBOT, Gap9551, Crzer07, LucienBOT, Vladimir Shmachkov, ZéroBot, Fredirib, Oracions, Dr Athanasis Boukalis, Lsparrish and Anonymous: 26

- **Lazarus sign** *Source:* https://en.wikipedia.org/wiki/Lazarus_sign?oldid=665051676 *Contributors:* Auric, Perceval, Rjwilmsi, Bedford, Pigman, BorgQueen, Olaf Davis, Nyttend, Grook Da Oger, Nono64, Alexbot, Addbot, Citation bot, Crzer07, Stiepan Pietrov, Ozzrhoads, Citation bot 1, I dream of horses, Todorb, Blotowij, Threefour15, RjwilmsiBot, Ctsinclair, Senator2029, Rockcenter, BattyBot and Anonymous: 11

- **Legal death** *Source:* https://en.wikipedia.org/wiki/Legal_death?oldid=661545493 *Contributors:* Scwlong, AnemoneProjectors, Niceguyedc, AnomieBOT, Srich32977, Cyberdog958, Miszatomic, Jim Carter, Oiyarbepsy and Anonymous: 2

- **Life support** *Source:* https://en.wikipedia.org/wiki/Life_support?oldid=688407058 *Contributors:* Ray Van De Walker, Patrick, Ixfd64, Karada, Paul A, Astudent, Heidimo, Saltine, Pakaran, Bearcat, David Gerard, Cobaltbluetony, Lupin, StargateX1, Rpyle731, Jfdwolff, Sesel, Hob, Erich gasboy, Antandrus, J3ff, Rich Farmbrough, Art LaPella, Weiwensg, Mytildebang, TACD, Wouterstomp, RainbowOfLight, Nuno Tavares, WCFrancis, Stevenfruitsmaak, Metropolitan90, WriterHound, Gaius Cornelius, Henryjimdix, Zzuuzz, JoanneB, Yvwv, SmackBot, YellowMonkey, Rhilsden, VMS Mosaic, Felix-felix, RomanSpa, Tifego, N2e, Cydebot, OrangutanCurse, Epbr123, Zé da Silva, Philippe, North Shoreman, Ingolfson, Albany NY, Boleslaw, Magioladitis, Bongwarrior, WhatamIdoing, Animum, MartinBot, Erasoft24, Pharaoh of the Wizards, Darth Gladius, Juliancolton, CardinalDan, Funandtrvl, VolkovBot, Z.E.R.O., Enviroboy, MCTales, Doc James, Main sister28, Flyer22 Reborn, Oxymoron83, Sanya3, Mygerardromance, ClueBot, SoCalDonF, Stupid2, Excirial, Jusdafax, Tnxman307, RexxS, Crazybrat, Addbot, Dawynn, Jncraton, Orange Carrot, Tide rolls, Lightbot, OlEnglish, Jarble, AVB, AnomieBOT, Rubinbot, Materialscientist, OllieFury, J04n, FrescoBot, Pinethicket, EmausBot, 19maxx, Ora Stendar, BrandonsLe, Brycehughes, ClueBot NG, Ypnypn, Widr, BG19bot, AlanPage007, ChrisGualtieri, Iamozy, Aymankamelwiki, Sbartl, Cook8530, Highway 231, Firebrace and Anonymous: 115

- **Locked-in syndrome** *Source:* https://en.wikipedia.org/wiki/Locked-in_syndrome?oldid=687946206 *Contributors:* The Anome, Fnielsen, Patrick, Taras, Delirium, Ahoerstemeier, TUF-KAT, Julesd, Triangular, Emperorbma, Furrykef, Nilmerg, Auric, Wolf530, Varlaam, Andycjp, Two Bananas, Joyous!, Bender235, Jarsyl, Dennis Brown, Renice, BarkingFish, Arcadian, KBi, Ivansanchez, Alansohn, TheParanoidOne, Arthena, Idont Havaname, Uucp, Linas, LOL, Guy M, GregorB, BD2412, Rjwilmsi, Quale, Fred Bradstadt, CloCkWeRX, Pumeleon, Stevenfruitsmaak, Diza, Ronebofh, Bgwhite, RussBot, Piet Delport, Varnav, Draeco, NawlinWiki, Sharik, MSJapan, Ccgrimm, Where next Columbus?, Rms125a@hotmail.com, Paul Erik, Groyolo, AndrewWTaylor, SmackBot, Profesh, Cubs Fan, NZUlysses, AndreasJS, Delldot, Chris the speller, Fuzzform, Simninja, Roscelese, Tekhnofiend, Scray, OSborn, Huon, Jumping cheese, Pwjb, Giancarlo Rossi, Dr. Crash, Salamurai, Deepred6502, Sbmehta, Scientizzle, Kashmiri, Jellonuts, Iska, SQGibbon, 5-HT8, Rezin8, Gregbard, Edward Hyde, The Photographer, Viciouslies, AniMate, Treybien, Asymptote, Anthonyhcole, Thijs!bot, Faigl.ladislav, Anupam, Headbomb, Trevyn, Dawkeye, Lunamaria, Steel breeze, Julia Rossi, AustinPowers69, Pinglis, SFairchild, Thylacinus cynocephalus, Albany NY, Awien, Rothorpe, Krguest, Wasell, Burhan Ahmed, Magioladitis, SHCarter, Froid, A3nm, Mikewhitcombe, Ariel., G-my, Ulkomaalainen, CFCF, Joebaum, Onhm, Willie the Walrein, Mikael Häggström, Brendan19, Olegwiki, BroJohnE, Bdixon, Thoroughbred Phoenix, CH52584, Cherryaa, Erik the Red 2, Salsera Aimee, Simonbowman9, Butterscotch, Joseph A. Spadaro, Doc James, Genni Seaton, Jesszahav, SieBot, Flyer22 Reborn, Oxymoron83, Ward20, Harel Newman, Hyperionsteel, Zer0431, SlackerMom, ClueBot, Mattgirling, Heracletus, Noxia, Songsmyth, XLinkBot, Koumz, Ost316, WillOakland, Airplaneman, Shallowdave, Addbot, Some jerk on the Internet, LeGagneur, DOI bot, Anwer Pasha, Download, 84user, Lightbot, OlEnglish, Legobot, Luckasbot, Yobot, JBains, EchetusXe, GateKeeper, AnomieBOT, Götz, Unara, Citation bot, SnorlaxMonster, LilHelpa, Cameron Scott, Xqbot, I Feel Tired, Gigemag76, Marcus1979, Firassalim, Tad Lincoln, Srich32977, Uhhhhhno, יעל12, Borsukers, Llib xoc, Fortdj33, RicHard-59, Medwed, Alexchen4836, TRATTOOO, Louperibot, Pinethicket, I dream of horses, Razorbelle, Dak1129, Jonesey95, SpaceFlight89, MJ, Superhands92, Proxtown, Tbhotch, Onel5969, RjwilmsiBot, EmausBot, Uniesert, Barzkar, Lucien504, Dadaist6174, Tommy2010, Wikipelli, Solomonfromfinland, ZéroBot, Bongoramsey, Ὁ οἶστρος, Onenone, Mariekemaus, PerimeterProf, Neil P. Quinn, SevenFound, Whoop whoop pull up, ClueBot NG, Flick33, Justlettersandnumbers, Pwduffy529, Nenesoccer14, Unautreadrien, Chocolate beans69, Frietjes, Widr, Lisaonlus, Helpful Pixie Bot, Newyork1501, Rockchalk717, Regulov, MicealWilson, YodaRULZ, BattyBot, CrunchySkies, YFdyh-bot, Gus Tuck, Swooncroon, Naturalspring, Jaffa507, CorrectItNow, Glenohumeral13, Michipedian, SamX, Larrywyse, Fitzcarmalan, Marandis, Ac3raven, Lorna Elwick, Valcanhouser, DrVentureWasRight, Monkbot, Filedelinkerbot, Fish storm, Imjohnho, LMBFam4, LavaBaron, Udahendi and Anonymous: 305

- **Mechanical ventilation** *Source:* https://en.wikipedia.org/wiki/Mechanical_ventilation?oldid=689365930 *Contributors:* AxelBoldt, Mav, Alex.tan, Rsabbatini, Patrick, Mahjongg, Kosebamse, Mkweise, Julesd, Tristanb, Samw, Quickbeam, Kat, Hydnjo, Wik, Zoicon5, Philb, Cdang, Chris Roy, Cdnc, Sverdrup, Hadal, Drstuey, Mcapdevila, Michael Devore, Jfdwolff, Beardo, Tom-, Erich gasboy, Chowbok, Sam Hocevar, Discospinster, Rich Farmbrough, Rama, Petersam, BjarteSorensen, Billlion, Mwanner, Arcadian, Me-tan, Pharos, Alansohn, Basie, Theaterfreak64, Wouterstomp, JoaoRicardo, Poromenos, Idont Havaname, Twisp, Gene Nygaard, Natalya, Richard Arthur Norton (1958-), Woohookitty, RHaworth, Tabletop, Dlauri, PeregrineAY, Mandarax, Graham87, Rjwilmsi, Old Moonraker, Stevenfruitsmaak, Koffieyahoo, Gaius Cornelius, InterwikiLinksRule, Nephron, Dissolve, Andrewr47, Caspian, Nescio, Elkman, Rwxrwxrwx, Cffrost, Lady BlahDeBlah, Alin0Steglinski, SmackBot, InvictaHOG, Delldot, TimBentley, RDBrown, Heliox00, A. B., DocJohnny, Metallurgist, Chrisirwin, Niels Olson, Mini-Geek, DMacks, -Marcus-, Andrewjuren, Gobonobo, Goodnightmush, Beetstra, Kyoko, P199, Acetylcholine, Hu12, JoeBot, ChrisCork, JForget, NickW557, Mwatg, Lightguy79, Calvero JP, Tetsu tmdu, Barticus88, Cyclonenim, AntiVandalBot, JAnDbot, MER-C, Magioladitis, Bdolcourt, JamesBWatson, Twsx, WhatamIdoing, Srice13, EagleFan, DerHexer, Yobol, Mmoneypenny, Nono64, Wiki Raja, FactsAndFigures, Mikael Häggström, Spinach Dip, Doctortomwiki, Tbone762, Bankhallbretherton, Whyso, Partha lal, Aesopos, Piggelin69~enwiki, Pfcpastry, RRT1107, V3development, Mariah24o7, Hallbrianh, Mendors, Countincr, Doc James, SieBot, Cl.crosby, Mike2vil, Ainlina, EoGuy, Mild Bill Hiccup, Piledhigheranddeeper, Chrisjw37, DumZiBoT, Rror, Kbdankbot, Addbot, Medicellis, Tide rolls, Yobot, Pliny82, Doudoumi, Gongshow, DiverDave, AnomieBOT, Piano non troppo, Citation bot, Honglindu, JmCor, J04n, RibotBOT, Mathonius, Pyjeon, FrescoBot, Paine Ellsworth, Mohshamy1976, India13, Pinethicket, A8UDI, Sahlan73, RedBot, Full-date unlinking bot, Kevinbowden, Arfgab, IMEwee, Ventilator63, MrArifnajafov, MAQUET Critical Care, Jackehammond, John of Reading, WikitanvirBot, RA0808, IbisHN, 28bot, ClueBot NG, Jeandédé, MelbourneStar, Helpful Pixie Bot, Appendinisapprentice, Je.rrt, Anesthsuperb, Atapapatom, NotWith, Pulmonological, Ayar5249, Cglion, EricEnfermero, BattyBot, Jethro B, SoledadKabocha, Mogism, Sriharsh1234, Asayari, Iztwoz, Eyesnore, Ddnegoita, Ashleyleia, Aeh.gmu, EtymAesthete, Monkbot, Crystallizedcarbon, Johanna, Gastroking, KasparBot, Lividsimone and Anonymous: 185

- **Minimally conscious state** *Source:* https://en.wikipedia.org/wiki/Minimally_conscious_state?oldid=684592821 *Contributors:* Janko, Radiojon, Viriditas, Arcadian, SlimVirgin, Mac Davis, Ruud Koot, Rjwilmsi, Bgwhite, Wavelength, Hairy Dude, Welsh, SmackBot, ScottHardie, Pwjb, Fig wright, Hu12, Amakuru, Cydebot, Awakennow, R'n'B, CommonsDelinker, Snikch, ElectricValkyrie, Master shepherd, Olegwiki, Pblaauw, 28bytes, Usrvoltaire, Neparis, ImageRemovalBot, GreekHouse, Niceguyedc, Addbot, Anwer Pasha, Mbinebri, Legobot, Rubinbot, Rjanag, Omnipaedista, Louperibot, Citation bot 1, Razorbelle, Trappist the monk, RjwilmsiBot, ElPeste, Ano593, Fæ, K kisses, MEDRS, BG19bot, Oliveralbq, DrunkSquirrel, Shin Andy Chung, ChrisGualtieri, Khazar2, Dexbot, Athomeinkobe, Anrnusna, Monkbot, SkateTier, Efthymios.angelakis and Anonymous: 21

- **Organ donation** *Source:* https://en.wikipedia.org/wiki/Organ_donation?oldid=689512120 *Contributors:* Lee Daniel Crocker, Vicki Rosenzweig, William Avery, Bdesham, Ihcoyc, Darkwind, Julesd, Glueball, Adam Conover, Feedmecereal, Wik, Zoicon5, Gakrivas, Pakaran, Shantavira, Fredrik, Kizor, Chris 73, Timrollpickering, Benc, Wile E. Heresiarch, McDutchie, Everyking, Jfdwolff, Eequor, Wmahan, OldakQuill, Fishal, Zhuuu, BozMo, Beland, CitoJam, EuroTom, Goh wz, Gscshoyru, Blue387, Imjustmatthew, Ukexpat, Ultrarob, Fuzlyssa, DMG413, Wikiti, Discospinster, Rich Farmbrough, Guanabot, Ffirehorse, Amicuspublilius, Inkypaws, Barista, TheWama, Mr. Billion, Wfisher, Aude, Remember, Giraffedata, Chirag, Kjkolb, Mareino, ADM, Alansohn, Anthony Appleyard, SlaveToTheWage, Arthena, Andrewpmk, Wouterstomp, Axl, Yummifruitbat, Ombudsman, Ashlux, Gible, PullUpYourSocks, Ceyockey, Dennis Bratland, Dismas, Mcsee, Bobrayner, Woohookitty, Dandv, Eleassar777, KevinOKeeffe, GregorB, Mandarax, Graham87, BD2412, Sjö, Rjwilmsi, SMC, Netan'el, Narcissus14, Bratch, FlaBot, Arnero, SouthernNights, Themanwithoutapast, Preslethe, Alphachimp, Chobot, DVdm, Tommylommykins, The Rambling Man, Ecemaml, Zafiroblue05, Salsb, Nahallac Silverwinds, Wiki alf, ONEder Boy, Mccready, Moe Epsilon, Kooky, DeadEyeArrow, Derek.cashman, Deville, Agapetos angel, Jules.LT, JWHPryor, Modify, GraemeL, Rathfelder, Teply, Paul Erik, Jeff Silvers, Alin0Steglinski, Jackafur, SmackBot, Eperotao, David Kernow, Hydrogen Iodide, C.Fred, Nil Einne, Edgar181, Malusmoriendumest, Gaff, Ohnoitsjamie, TimBentley, BarkerJr, Atomsprengja, MalafayaBot, SchfiftyThree, Deli nk, Kevin Ryde, Nbarth, Sgt Pinback, Davidcohen, Can't sleep, clown will eat me, Shuki, Rludlow, JonHarder, Mokeyboy, Vyxx, Daveundis, Jackohare, Lisasmall, Sigma 7, Kukini, Ohconfucius, SashatoBot, ArglebargleIV, Kuru, General Ization, Heimstern, SilkTork, Gobonobo, Mr. Vernon, Stupid Corn, Mr Stephen, Kyoko, Biwhite2, Arstchnca, Bwpach, Hu12, Balkissoonsingh, Kencf0618, Billtheking, Kal1917, Twas Now, Chovain, Ceochris, Dev920, JForget, Melicans, Gregbard, JVinocur, Cydebot, Reywas92, Anthonyhcole, Myscrnnm, Tawkerbot4, Lightguy79, Chrislk02, Emmett5, Thijs!bot, RapidR, Silver seren, Genpark, Myanw, Ioeth, Papa Ben, Jimmy, SiobhanHansa, Bob smith6968, Magioladitis, VoABot II, Bequw, Glasshutch, Catgut, WhatamIdoing, Allstarecho, Mjwoolf, WLU, Oroso, James JK, Sasper, Anaxial, D Dinneen, Pbroks13, Lilac Soul, Marcusmax, McSly, Mikael Häggström, Skier Dude, InspectorTiger, Ktsparkman, Juliancolton, Cometstyles, Deor, VolkovBot, One GG, Alchemystical, Oshwah, Vipinhari, Miranda, Maxkin, Cesano, Oxfordwang, Jackfork, Bearian, Unoluigi, Cgperry, Blurpeace, Dirkbb, Teh roflmaoer, Purgatory Fubar, Bsayusd, Seraphita~enwiki, Hayyimdanzig,

Legoktm, SieBot, Tiddly Tom, Jauerback, VVVBot, Mangostar, Flyer22 Reborn, Radon210, Oxymoron83, Nanophys, Svick, Fuddle, Wabbit98, Florentino floro, Missyagogo, ClueBot, FoxDiamond, Binksternet, Badger Drink, DonateLife, Jan1nad, Unbuttered Parsnip, Freebullets, Rglater, CounterVandalismBot, Niceguyedc, Gnome de plume, Hi123987, Lartoven, Camerajohn, Razorflame, Atomic811, La Pianista, Anonrocker, DumZiBoT, XLinkBot, Stickee, RJ Transplant, Mitch Ames, Mifter, Mahlonslee, Addbot, Cjneversleeps, Willking1979, Jafeluv, Comanox, Micromaster, Hda3ku, GSMR, Blethering Scot, MrOllie, Download, Lihaas, Holeymoleytoad102, Cactus8227, Beachdude2k, Tide rolls, Lightbot, Zorrobot, Legobot, Luckas-bot, Yobot, Legobot II, Freikorp, DiverDave, AnomieBOT, Thuvan Dihn, Azmansell, Materialscientist, 90 Auto, Triumph of the Bill, Citation bot, OllieFury, ArthurBot, Obersachsebot, Jsharpminor, Ruby.red.roses, J04n, ODTF, Omnipaedista, Wiki1010101, Xanatos290, Uhhhhhno, Shadowjams, Dougofborg, BloodGrapefruit2, FrescoBot, Kelsey399, Astronomyinertia, Welshsocialist, Cannolis, Descemet, Pinethicket, Jonesey95, Triplestop, RedBot, Serols, ஜெ.மொழிச்செல்வி, Σ, Vaerinne, Plasticspork, ReneeFeltz, Venujustforu, Vikram2rhyme, Natausha07, Bbarkley2, Californiafixer, Lotje, Vrenator, TBloemink, Suffusion of Yellow, Reach Out to the Truth, Vijayakumarblathur, DARTH SIDIOUS 2, RjwilmsiBot, Wintonian, Grondemar, EmausBot, John of Reading, RA0808, Arroz75, Tommy2010, K6ka, ZéroBot, Bollyjeff, Doddy Wuid, Jake603, H3llBot, L Kensington, Gsarwa, Seniorexpat, Pigfarmer65, Cornell92, Bill william compton, Sven Manguard, DASHBotAV, DemonicPartyHat, E. Fokker, Will Beback Auto, ClueBot NG, YellowAries2010, Satellizer, Cdbradley, Widr, Helpful Pixie Bot, Connorrosenbeck, BG19bot, Megjones01, KateWishing, PhnomPencil, RandomLettersForName, SStidsen, Adiroth, Snow Blizzard, MrBill3, Stimulieconomy, Johnny locks sudbury, Gampa1111, TBrandley, Achowat, Geeksnglitter, Pratyya Ghosh, Stevewpbfl, Cyberbot II, ChrisGualtieri, Mogism, Lugia2453, SFK2, OrganFacts, KenHiggs, Andyhowlett, Boydchandler378457587, NathanWubs, Laurencasebolt, Jodosma, ArmbrustBot, Kharkiv07, Ugog Nizdast, Sue Gianstefani, AioftheStorm, Quenhitran, Keepinternetfree, Praveenrajan27, JenTintheD, Robevans123, JaconaFrere, Gryne, Castroregu, Krishnatasha, Monkbot, Ca2james, Kwaldby10, Scarlettail, Amortias, Lullabye49, Lythronaxargestes, Claw10566, Poiuytrewqvtaatv123321, AthenaEleven, BT80, Agroppe21, Catstan95, Brigidmcfarland, KasparBot, Melizkell, Dereksudduth, Niko kirito, Deekshit bunny and Anonymous: 511

- **Persistent vegetative state** *Source:* https://en.wikipedia.org/wiki/Persistent_vegetative_state?oldid=682404686 *Contributors:* The Anome, Ed Poor, Amillar, Alex.tan, Patrick, Michael Hardy, Kroose, Karada, NuclearWinner, Plop, Kingturtle, Irmgard, Janko, WhisperToMe, Tpbradbury, Omegatron, SD6-Agent, Robbot, Kizor, Schutz, Altenmann, Psychonaut, Nurg, Postdlf, Apol0gies, Frencheigh, Jfdwolff, AlistairMcMillan, Gyrofrog, Chowbok, Loremaster, Capnned, Joyous!, Jcw69, GreenReaper, Adashiel, Kate, Mike Rosoft, Chris Howard, Freakofnurture, Johncapistrano, Rich Farmbrough, Bender235, Cyclopia, Diogenes~enwiki, S.K., Petersam, FirstPrinciples, Lankiveil, Thickslab, Grick, John Vandenberg, Viriditas, Arcadian, Kbir1, Eruantalon, Pontifex, Alansohn, Anthony Appleyard, Gargaj, Eric Kvaalen, Primalchaos, AzaToth, SlimVirgin, Hondje~enwiki, Forteblast, Johnwcowan, JAL, Stuartyeates, Woohookitty, LOL, Guy M, Sellario, Before My Ken, Urod, Tabletop, Cloaked Romulan, Grace Note, Eaolson, Isnow, Aidje, NCdave, BD2412, Powergrid, Rjwilmsi, Seraphimblade, A ghost, Yamamoto Ichiro, Fish and karate, FlaBot, VKokielov, SchuminWeb, Tropix, MSDOJD, Alphachimp, GordonWatts, Introvert, Chobot, YurikBot, Err0neous, Ihope127, Nrets, Raven4x4x, MSJapan, Syrthiss, Mysid, Nikkimaria, Tevildo, Paul Erik, AndrewWTaylor, SmackBot, Delldot, Sardino, Apers0n, Brianski, Master of Puppets, Papa November, Stevage, The Rogue Penguin, EOZyo, Maxt, Jaimie Henry, Mistamagic28, Mtmelendez, Pwjb, Maxwahrhaftig, WereWolf, Giancarlo Rossi, Paul KMK, Scientizzle, SilkTork, Robofish, Joffeloff, Filippowiki, Vjhenderson, Pedantic of Purley, MrArt, Fluppy, Ra5ul, Brufiki, SimonD, Hydra Rider, Ecco1983, B-D, JForget, VoxLuna, Dycedarg, CBM, Gregbard, Cydebot, Michaelas10, Lugnuts, Pustelnik, CieloEstrellado, StarGeek, SeNeKa, Headbomb, Nick Number, Dovea, AntiVandalBot, Sun Tzu Eraserhead, Seaphoto, Farosdaughter, Kauczuk, Falconleaf, Fshafique, Barek, OhanaUnited, Magioladitis, Grobbman22, Nyttend, Cartoon Boy, Zebraic, EagleFan, David Eppstein, Tins128, Tinmanic, Scottalter, Yobol, R'n'B, AstroHurricane001, Dalton40, V22arvind, Plasticup, Belovedfreak, NewEnglandYankee, Jmodum90, Mlle thenardier, VolkovBot, Vlmastra, Martinevans123, Thycid, Steven J. Anderson, LeaveSleaves, LiquidEyes, Tomaxer, Js8391a, Doc James, AlleborgoBot, Neparis, Brenont, SiegeLord, Sammyk214, Steven Crossin, Tripod86, Martarius, ClueBot, The Thing That Should Not Be, Coralmizu, NatalieGerblick, 7&6=thirteen, M.O.X, Doprendek, Bathis, Thingg, Dana boomer, Londonclanger, Liberal Humanist, HD86, Jes roo, Jytdog, Avoided, Airplaneman, Farkoff, Samiam1611, EEng, Zolstijers, Addbot, American Eagle, RPHv, DOI bot, Thabizzness, Anwer Pasha, Looie496, MrOllie, Download, Bwrs, Tide rolls, Lightbot, OlEnglish, Pietrow, Luckas-bot, Yobot, Nallimbot, AnomieBOT, IncidentalPoint, Citation bot, Opinions, ArthurBot, Quebec99, Obersachsebot, Xqbot, Bugs2012, Ethics2med, Headlikeawhole, Tyrol5, Srich32977, Anonymous from the 21st century, GrouchoBot, GorgeCustersSabre, GenOrl, Et bravo, BloodGrapefruit2, FrescoBot, Pepper, Stephen Morley, Citation bot 1, Razorbelle, Mmjeae, Laureys1, Trappist the monk, Dinamik-bot, WhatGuy, Wilytilt, EmausBot, Grammarz, -- -- --, Barzkar, Djembayz, H3llBot, AManWithNoPlan, OnePt618, MaryFrancisK, Cbaltes, SBaker43, Ego White Tray, HandsomeFella, BabbaQ, Whoop whoop pull up, ClueBot NG, Danishcanadian, Snotbot, Humbugling, MEDRS, Carlstak, Cranmills, SLMnovelli, Neurotrope, Art348, YFdyh-bot, JYBot, CasparRH, Frosty, SomeFreakOnTheInternet, PurserSmith, Hamoudafg, Flyingtoast, Egocentrix, Nauriya, Bali88, Monkbot, Graptoscan, Sckayv2.2, 400 Lux, Miranda Close, Bobmcfred45, Heavengemini and Anonymous: 234

- **Pupillary reflex** *Source:* https://en.wikipedia.org/wiki/Pupillary_reflex?oldid=675801471 *Contributors:* Carlossuarez46, Bearcat, Xezbeth, Arcadian, JForget, Hordaland, Jusdafax, AnomieBOT, BG19bot and Anonymous: 5

- **Unconsciousness** *Source:* https://en.wikipedia.org/wiki/Unconsciousness?oldid=676470863 *Contributors:* The Anome, Robert Brook, Youandme, Patrick, Michael Hardy, Sannse, 5ko, Julesd, Like a Virgin, Robbot, Wolfkeeper, Zigger, Wicked~enwiki, Erich gasboy, Lacrimosus, Rfl, MBisanz, Shanes, Arcadian, Cavrdg, Sheehan, Echuck215, Markaci, BD2412, Yurik, Amire80, FlaBot, Rysz, Alphachimp, Manufracture, David91, Stephenb, Mysid, NWalker, SmackBot, Gilliam, Bluebot, COMPFUNK2, Vasiliy Faronov, Rukario639, Bjankuloski06en~enwiki, 16@r, Ex nihil, DabMachine, SweetNeo85, Billyb~enwiki, Storkk, Colin MacLaurin, JAnDbot, Magioladitis, JamesBWatson, Scottalter, Fusion7, Nullie, Sasajid, MariaNewman, Master shepherd, Vanished user 39948282, Jarry1250, Joutsen-DD, D6chung, Shouriki, ScAvenger lv, UB65, Kjramesh, Vanisheduser12345, Razorflame, Editor2020, Imagine Reason, Vanished user oerjio4kdm3, Legobot, TaBOT-zerem, EricWester, Rubinbot, James500, Xqbot, Machine Elf 1735, Pinethicket, EmausBot, أحمد مصطفى السيد, Tisane, Sepguilherme, ClueBot NG, PhnomPencil, BattyBot, ChrisGualtieri, Everything Is Numbers, Martinedezoete and Anonymous: 47

- **Uniform Determination of Death Act** *Source:* https://en.wikipedia.org/wiki/Uniform_Determination_of_Death_Act?oldid=687265955 *Contributors:* The Anome, Emperorbma, HorsePunchKid, Neutrality, Cburnett, RJFJR, PullUpYourSocks, BD2412, Koavf, AntiSpamBot, Skeptic06, Oschroeder, PigFlu Oink, Alex Capron and Anonymous: 10

- **Vegetative symptoms** *Source:* https://en.wikipedia.org/wiki/Vegetative_symptoms?oldid=624495900 *Contributors:* Michael Hardy, Gccwang, Supten, SmackBot, Bluebot, RDBrown, Cydebot, Jamie Lokier, Mattisse, Niceguyedc, 1ForTheMoney, FiachraByrne, Monkbot and Anonymous: 1

- **Vestibulo–ocular reflex** *Source:* https://en.wikipedia.org/wiki/Vestibulo%E2%80%93ocular_reflex?oldid=659301813 *Contributors:* The Anome, Infrogmation, Corixidae, Selket, Saltine, Cyberied, Eequor, Mporch, Arcadian, Davidljung, Guy M, Dolfrog, Firien, BD2412, Rjwilmsi,

3.2 Images

- **File:Scotland_DNACPR_-_obverse.png** *Source:* https://upload.wikimedia.org/wikipedia/commons/6/61/Scotland_DNACPR_-_obverse. png *License:* OGL *Contributors:* http://www.scotland.gov.uk/Publications/2010/05/24095633/15 *Original artist:* Scottish Government

- **File:Simple_vestibulo-ocular_reflex.PNG** *Source:* https://upload.wikimedia.org/wikipedia/commons/5/58/Simple_vestibulo-ocular_reflex. PNG *License:* CC-BY-SA-3.0 *Contributors:* Image:ThreeNeuronArc.png *Original artist:* User:Mikael Häggström

- **File:Symbol_list_class.svg** *Source:* https://upload.wikimedia.org/wikipedia/en/d/db/Symbol_list_class.svg *License:* Public domain *Contributors:* ? *Original artist:* ?

- **File:Unbalanced_scales.svg** *Source:* https://upload.wikimedia.org/wikipedia/commons/f/fe/Unbalanced_scales.svg *License:* Public domain *Contributors:* ? *Original artist:* ?

- **File:VIP_Bird2.jpg** *Source:* https://upload.wikimedia.org/wikipedia/commons/9/94/VIP_Bird2.jpg *License:* Public domain *Contributors:* Own work *Original artist:* Brian Hall

- **File:Vestibulo-ocular_reflex_EN.svg** *Source:* https://upload.wikimedia.org/wikipedia/commons/8/84/Vestibulo-ocular_reflex_EN.svg *License:* GFDL *Contributors:* own work, based on Image:Simple_vestibulo-ocular_reflex.PNG and Image:ThreeNeuronArc.png *Original artist:* .Koen

- **File:Virginia_Sample_DDNR.jpg** *Source:* https://upload.wikimedia.org/wikipedia/en/0/00/Virginia_Sample_DDNR.jpg *License:* ? *Contributors:*
  http://www.vdh.virginia.gov/OEMS/Files_Page/DDNR/DDNRSample.pdf *Original artist:*
  Commonwealth of Virginia

- **File:Wiki_letter_w_cropped.svg** *Source:* https://upload.wikimedia.org/wikipedia/commons/1/1c/Wiki_letter_w_cropped.svg *License:* CC-BY-SA-3.0 *Contributors:*

- Wiki_letter_w.svg *Original artist:* Wiki_letter_w.svg: Jarkko Piiroinen

- **File:Wiktionary-logo-en.svg** *Source:* https://upload.wikimedia.org/wikipedia/commons/f/f8/Wiktionary-logo-en.svg *License:* Public domain *Contributors:* Vector version of Image:Wiktionary-logo-en.png. *Original artist:* Vectorized by Fvasconcellos (talk · contribs), based on original logo tossed together by Brion Vibber

3.3　Content license

Made in the USA
Coppell, TX
06 September 2021

61873768R00057